1982

W9-BQM-077

Principles of quality assurance

3 0301 00068171 4

A publication of the
Association of American Medical Colleges

Principles of Quality Assurance and Cost Containment in Health Care

A Guide for Medical Students,
Residents, and Other Health Professionals

John W. Williamson, M.D.
James I. Hudson, M.D.
Madeline M. Nevins, Ph.D.

Principles of Quality Assurance and Cost Containment in Health Care

LIBRARY
College of St. Francis
JOLIET, ILL.

Jossey-Bass Publishers

San Francisco • Washington • London • 1982

PRINCIPLES OF QUALITY ASSURANCE AND COST CONTAINMENT IN HEALTH CARE
A Guide for Medical Students, Residents, and Other Health Professionals
by John W. Williamson, James I. Hudson, and Madeline M. Nevins

Copyright © 1982 by: Association of American
                        Medical Colleges
                        One Dupont Circle, Suite 200
                        Washington, D.C. 20036

                        Jossey-Bass Inc., Publishers
                        433 California Street
                        San Francisco, California 94104

                        Jossey-Bass Limited
                        28 Banner Street
                        London EC1Y 8QE

Copyright under International, Pan American, and
Universal Copyright Conventions. All rights
reserved. No part of this book may be reproduced
in any form—except for brief quotation (not to
exceed 1,000 words) in a review or professional
work—without permission in writing from the publishers.

Library of Congress Cataloging in Publication Data

Williamson, John W.
        Principles of quality assurance and cost containment in health care.

        (Association of American Medical Colleges series in academic
medicine)
        Bibliography: p. 129
        Includes index.
        1. Medical care—Quality control.
2. Medical care—Cost control. I. Hudson, James I. II. Nevins, Madeline
M. III. Title. IV. Series. [DNLM. 1. Quality assurance, Health
care—United States. 2. Cost control. W 84 W65p]
RA399.A1W545   1982   362.1   82-48072
ISBN 0-87589-531-X

Manufactured in the United States of America

The paper in this book meets the guidelines for
permanence and durability of the Committee on
Production Guidelines for Book Longevity of the
Council on Library Resources.

JACKET DESIGN BY WILLI BAUM

FIRST EDITION

Code 8224

G
362.1
W936p

The Jossey-Bass Series
in Higher Education

ݓݓݓݓݓݓݓݓݓݓݓݓݓݓݓݓݓݓݓݓݓݓ

Association of American Medical Colleges
Series in Academic Medicine
JOHN A.D. COOPER, *Editor*

102669

Contents

ﭏﭏﭏﭏﭏﭏﭏﭏﭏﭏﭏﭏﭏﭏﭏﭏﭏﭏﭏﭏﭏﭏﭏﭏﭏﭏﭏﭏﭏﭏﭏﭏ

Foreword

๙๙๙๙๙๙๙๙๙๙๙๙๙๙๙๙๙๙๙๙๙๙๙๙๙

This volume and its companion piece, *Teaching Quality Assurance and Cost Containment in Health Care: A Faculty Guide,* the first two publications in the Association of American Medical Colleges' Series on Academic Medicine, respond to growing concerns about the quality of medical care and its escalating costs. Together they provide an auspicious debut for the series, which will examine major issues in the administration and conduct of medical education.

The growing complexity of medical care—as well as the rapidity with which new knowledge from the research laboratories is increasing the effectiveness of prevention, diagnosis, and therapy—makes it increasingly important to assure that patients are receiving care of high quality. An important aspect of quality medical care is the appropriate use of the new techniques and technologies available to the physician. Overuse is not compatible with high quality or with the need to contain costs in an era of diminishing resources for medical care.

John Williamson and his coauthors are recognized authorities in the field of quality assurance and cost containment. The two volumes were based on a series of workshops sponsored by the Association of American Medical Colleges and designed to introduce quality assurance and cost containment into medical education. The materials were modified on the basis of field tests at selected sites by medical school faculty, students, and residents.

This guide for medical students, residents, and other health professionals outlines the five stages of quality assurance that encompass cost containment principles. More importantly, it uses illustrative case histories and a problem-solving approach that are directly applicable to the educational setting and in clinical practice. Unlike more theoretical works on the subject, it is organized so that students and health professionals can actually learn to apply theory to practice. It is a valuable contribution in responding to the growing consensus about the importance of including such material in the curriculum of health professional education.

Principles of Quality Assurance and Cost Containment will serve several needs. Faculty and students will find that it responds to the need for a book in formal instructional programs. Others will find it useful as a resource for incorporating quality assurance and cost containment into the basic clinical sciences. For individual health professionals who are seeking to enhance their personal commitment to the principles of quality assurance and cost containment, it will serve as a valuable self-instructional tool. The usefulness of this book is not restricted to medical students and young physicians. Serious individuals in other health professions with patient care responsibilities will find the book equally valuable.

It is clear that in an era of restricted resources and expanding technologies for medical care, increased attention must be paid to containing costs. There is a corollary requirement that the highest possible care be provided within the restrictions imposed. This volume will help physicians and other health professionals respond to this important challenge.

July 1982   John A.D. Cooper, M.D., Ph.D.
President, Association of
American Medical Colleges

Preface

꒜꒜꒜꒜꒜꒜꒜꒜꒜꒜꒜꒜꒜꒜꒜꒜꒜꒜꒜꒜꒜꒜꒜꒜

The terms *quality assurance* and *cost containment* appear not only in current medical literature but also in the front pages of daily newspapers, in articles published in popular weekly magazines, in major political speeches, and in federal legislation. The increasing frequency with which these issues are discussed indicates that concern about quality and cost of medical care has become a matter of national importance that will profoundly influence the present and future practice of medical care. This guide answers some basic questions that arise in connection with the discussion of quality assurance and cost containment, questions such as:

- What do quality assurance and cost containment mean, and why are members of the medical profession concerned with these issues?

- What does one need to know about quality assurance and cost containment in order to incorporate them into the practice of medical care?
- How does one go about conducting a study of the quality and cost of care?
- Where are the data needed to conduct such studies?

Chapter One presents the rationale for learning about quality assurance and places the issue in a historical perspective. Chapters Two and Three explain the basic concepts that must be understood in conducting quality assurance and cost containment studies. These chapters are supplemented by appendixes containing sources of national and local data for each concept. The fourth chapter outlines the five stages of a quality assurance and cost containment study, illustrating each stage by means of an actual case study of quality and costs.

In this text, quality and cost of care are viewed as inextricably intertwined. Consequently, the term *quality assurance* is used to refer to assessment and improvement of the effect of care *and* of the way resources are utilized to provide that care. In other words, we will use the term *quality assurance* to encompass what has been traditionally called quality (that is, effectiveness) of care *and* what is currently implied by "cost containment" (that is, efficiency). In fact, whenever the term *cost containment* appears in these pages it is intended to make explicit the second dimension of the definition of quality assurance—namely, the assessment and improvement in resource utilization (or efficiency)—and it does not carry the narrow connotation of reduction in charges.

Besides comprehending the meaning of quality assurance as used in this text, readers must understand that the approach described is mainly applied to measuring the effectiveness and efficiency of care provided to a given aggregate population in a specific setting by a group of providers within a given institution (for example, group practice, hospital, long-term care facility). This does not mean that the principles and methods discussed in the text do not apply to the assessment and improvement of care provided to individual patients. However, it does recognize the difficulties inherent in attempting to assess and improve every aspect of care provided to every patient, and it suggests that the most efficient way of improving individual patient care derives from identifying the problems that affect a large portion of the patient population. Identification of and improvement in such problem areas will necessarily improve the care of individual patients as well.

The process of conducting a quality assurance study is much like the process used in clinical management of a patient. To demonstrate how closely the one parallels the other, it might be useful to draw an analogy between clinical problem solving and quality assurance in terms of the types of information they require and the decision-making process they use.

Clinical Problem Solving. A physician follows certain basic steps in managing a patient. First, an initial work-up (including a history, physical examination, and perhaps a few screening laboratory tests) is performed to develop a priority list of conditions to be explored. To do this well, two types of information are needed: that provided by the patient in terms of clinical findings and that possessed by the physician on health conditions to which these findings might relate. Second, specific clinical data are sought to confirm or rule out high-priority, hypothesized problems. Third, a differential diagnosis is formulated and additional data obtained to establish a more definitive diagnosis, including problem etiology and treatment considerations necessary to develop a therapeutic plan. As part of this therapeutic planning, the physician will undoubtedly make some cost-effectiveness decisions, perhaps intuitively. Fourth, the physician implements the therapeutic plan thus formulated. Finally, a procedure is established to evaluate the treatment provided (for example, follow-up visit, telephone report) and to plan further action if required.

The Quality Assurance Process. Quality assurance studies follow the same stages as clinical management, and similar types of information are required for each stage. In this instance, however, the "patient" with the presenting problem is an aggregate group of both patients and providers within an office or institutional health care setting, while the "provider" is the quality assurance team. The team proceeds much as the clinical provider does. A priority list of problems amenable to improvement is developed and problems for study selected. This step is analogous to the first stage in patient management—the development of a list of conditions to be explored based on the initial work-up. At this stage of quality assurance study, the team needs information on the importance of perceived problems (such as frequency of occurrence and costs), on the efficacy of available interventions, on the likely current efficiency and effectiveness of the health care now provided, and on the potential for achieving improvement if deficiency is documented. Second, for any given high-priority problem, the team completes an initial assessment study to confirm or rule out that problem. This process is similar to the focused data gathering and problem confirmation of patient management. Third, the team must make a definitive assessment of the nature of the problem in order to identify problem causes (etiology) and considerations needed to develop a specific action plan to achieve the desired improvement—a process analogous to formulating a differential diagnosis, establishing a final diagnosis, and planning therapy in patient management. Fourth, the improvement plan is then implemented, just as, in patient management, treatment is prescribed and carried out. Finally, the team assesses the results of the study to determine to what extent the desired improvement was realized, a step similar to patient follow-up in clinical management.

With these definitions and similarities in mind, we can now examine why physicians need to know about quality assurance and cost containment, what they must learn, and how they can use quality assurance and cost containment studies to improve the care they provide.

August 1982

John W. Williamson
Boston, Massachusetts

James I. Hudson
Utrecht, The Netherlands

Madeline M. Nevins
Washington, D.C.

Acknowledgments

𝕶𝕶𝕶𝕶𝕶𝕶𝕶𝕶𝕶𝕶𝕶𝕶𝕶𝕶𝕶𝕶𝕶𝕶𝕶𝕶𝕶𝕶𝕶

The preparation of this text was made possible by a grant from the Health Care Financing Administration (Grant No. 18-P-97124/3-01) to the Department of Health Services of the Association of American Medical Colleges and the School of Hygiene and Public Health of the Johns Hopkins University. Much of the material in this text was originally prepared for use in *Teaching Quality Assurance and Cost Containment in Health Care: A Faculty Guide,* the companion volume to this book. The approach, as well as the fundamental principles of quality assurance on which this text is based, is the work of John W. Williamson, the principal author of the faculty resource. The information on efficacy and its application to quality assurance was contributed by Daniel M. Barr; the information on health care costs was developed by Mary Lee Ingbar; Jay Noren contributed the material on effectiveness and efficiency; and William F. Jessee is responsible for the information on achieving improvement. Material on curriculum development prepared by Mohan L. Garg, Donald R. Korst, and Frank T. Stritter has been incorporated into this text, as has the history of quality assurance developed by Elizabeth Fee.

The authors and editors are particularly grateful to the medical school students, residents, and faculty who participated in the field testing of the original manuscript and whose recommendations led to the development of this separate text for students and residents. It would be impossible to name all faculty and students who participated in the field testing of this material. However, special thanks are due to the following faculty who acted as coordinators at the field test sites: C. M. G. Buttery, associate professor of community medicine, Department of Family Medicine, Eastern Virginia Medical School; Herbert Lukashok, associate professor and acting chairman, Department of Community Health, Albert Einstein College of Medicine, Yeshiva University; Kathleen Morton, deputy director of Ambulatory Services, Montefiore Hospital and Medical Center; Joseph Gonnella, associate dean and director of Academic Programs, and Carter Zeleznik, associate director of the Offices of Medical Education, Jefferson Medical College, Thomas Jefferson University; William M. Marine, director of the Department of Preventive Medicine and Comprehensive Health Care, University of Colorado School of Medicine; Michael J. Garland, assistant professor, Department of Public Health, University of Oregon Health Science Center; Louise Ball, special assistant to the dean, and Samuel C. Matheny, Division of Family Medicine, University of Southern California School of Medicine; Charles Begley, assistant professor, Department of Medical Humanities, Southern Illinois University School of Medicine; and Herman S. Wigodsky, clinical professor, Department of Pathology, University of Texas Health Science Center at San Antonio.

A final word of thanks is extended to Dian Nelson and Katherine Hubscher, project secretaries in the Department of Health Services at the Association of American Medical Colleges, and to Bernice F. Culp, secretary to the Department of Health Services Administration at the Johns Hopkins University.

The Authors

❧❧❧❧❧❧❧❧❧❧❧❧❧❧❧❧❧❧❧❧❧❧❧❧❧❧❧❧

John W. Williamson is visiting professor of international health, Department of Biostatistics, Harvard School of Public Health, and on leave from the School of Hygiene and Public Health, Johns Hopkins University.

James I. Hudson is staff member, National Organization for Quality Assessment in Hospitals, Utrecht, The Netherlands.

Madeline M. Nevins is staff associate, Association of American Medical Colleges.

Renate Wilson, who served as coordinating editor on this book, is research associate at the School of Hygiene and Public Health, Johns Hopkins University, and editorial associate at the National Center for Health Services Research.

Principles of Quality Assurance and Cost Containment in Health Care

A Guide for Medical Students, Residents, and Other Health Professionals

The Importance of Quality Assurance and Cost Containment in Current Health Care

ᴕᴕᴕᴕᴕᴕᴕᴕᴕᴕᴕᴕᴕᴕᴕᴕᴕᴕᴕᴕᴕᴕᴕᴕᴕ

A number of societal problems and values are presently influenc- ing the health care delivery system. Taken together, they provide a rationale for learning quality assurance and cost containment and applying it at all levels of this system. The American public has grown increasingly concerned with the quality of care. This con- cern is reflected in questions raised about the efficacy of certain common medical procedures, in debates over the harmful side ef- fects of widely prescribed drugs, and in inquiries into the necessity of frequently performed surgical procedures. The results of this concern are evident in the growth of self-help groups that spurn the services of the health care delivery system and turn to natural remedies for treating illness, in the increase in number of malprac- tice suits, in the frequent references to iatrogenic illnesses, and in the proliferation of federal programs to monitor and assess the efficacy and safety of new medical technologies and drugs.

1

An equal degree of concern is apparent with respect to costs of medical care. The media abound with reports about the rising costs of medical care and the subsequent effect on federal spending and insurance costs. These reports raise questions about the increasing discrepancy between available resources and the exponential growth in the cost of medical care. Concern is expressed about the just allocation of medical care resources and the danger of exhausting the supply of, or the ability and willingness to pay for, these resources in the future. Hiatt, at Harvard University, applying Hardin's concept of the tragedy of the commons to the total resources available for medical care, identifies three current medical practices that endanger the future availability of medical resources: (1) doing everything possible for the individual patient regardless of the risks or benefits to society at large, (2) expending resources on health care interventions that benefit neither the individual nor society, and (3) applying highly technological medical interventions to attempt to cure conditions that could be prevented by less costly means (Hiatt, 1975). To these practices must be added the fact that additional demands will be made on the available supply of medical resources as the population ages and as attempts are made to correct current inadequacies in care for large sectors of the population.

Response to this concern over costs and availability of resources has taken many forms—from voluntary efforts by physicians and hospitals to control costs to the establishment of federal agencies to review the appropriateness of health care expenditures. Effective quality assurance cost containment programs are another way of responding to these societal concerns about quality and cost. By proposing to improve the effectiveness and efficiency with which care is delivered, they offer one approach to resolving the societal value conflict inherent in consumer demand for more resources and improved quality of care and the concomitant insistence on controlling costs.

A second rationale for learning how to conduct quality assurance and cost containment studies springs from the demands placed on practicing physicians by their colleagues and peers. For some time, the medical profession has tried to ensure that quality care would be provided by accrediting training programs and care facilities, certifying physicians, and requiring continuing medical education. More recently some professional societies have begun to require recertification to ensure that their members retain their knowledge and skills as well as keep abreast of new developments in medical care (American Board of Medical Specialties, 1979).

Most recently attempts have been made to incorporate into various accreditation procedures an assessment of individual and institutional abilities to conduct quality assurance and cost containment studies (Joint Commission on Accreditation of Hospitals, 1979). The Joint Commission on Accreditation of Hospitals (JCAH) has developed a program to assist hospitals to meet the quality assurance requirement contained in the JCAH accreditation procedures, and it has been suggested that questions on quality assurance and cost containment be included in the board examination for all specialties. From the beginning Professional Standards Review Organizations (PSROs) have recommended linkage of continuing medical education programs within the hospital to problems identified during PSRO studies. Within the last year, the *New England Journal of Medicine* published an article advocating that performance review, which has the support of the American Society of Internal Medicine, be adopted as the most direct appraisal of physician competence in both hospital and outpatient settings (Farrington, Felch, and Hare, 1980).

Given the increasing importance attached to quality assurance and cost containment by the medical profession itself, it is apparent that future physicians need to learn the essentials of quality assurance and to develop a professional attitude toward continual self-assessment and lifelong learning. Participation in peer review, quality assurance, and cost containment activities as well as study of basic concepts and procedures during the years of professional training will develop the requisite knowledge and skills for carrying out future professional responsibilities in these areas.

In addition to the reasons based on societal demands and professional requirements, there is a more intrinsic rationale for learning about quality assurance and cost containment: the need of providers to be certain that the care provided meets their standards of excellence. Later in this text, data will be provided on the most common ambulatory and short-stay hospital health problems.

These data show that often the physician will be dealing with asymptomatic patients or with nonserious illnesses (for example, sore throats, colds, and "flu") that are frequently self-limiting and require routine management (for example, bed rest, fluids, and aspirin). Such problems can become a source of frustration, if not professional "burnout," to the provider who approaches practice with the belief that all health problems will be "interesting" and therapeutically challenging. Faced with difficulties of non-compliance and multiple health problems resulting as much from socioeconomic and life-style conditions as from disease, the individual provider needs to know how to evaluate his or her work to be assured that the true nature of the problem is understood and that appropriate action is being taken. This may require going beyond the diagnosis of the illness to identify ways of improving health outcomes, patient satisfaction, and efficient delivery of care. Early training in the problem identification and decision-making processes associated with quality assurance and cost containment can forestall physician frustration and dissatisfaction by alerting future physicians to other components of delivering health care, such as education of patients and sensitivity to patients' life situations, that will make future practice more satisfying.

This training will also develop a sense of personal accountability for health care costs. Increasingly the public is asking the individual physician to be aware of his or her role in increasing the costs of health care and to consider the broader social implications resulting from depletion of available resources. If medical school curricula and residency programs contain components on methods of evaluating both the quality and costs of care, future physicians will be better able to respond to this public demand for accountability.

History of the Current Mandate for Quality Assurance

The preceding section described what may be called the intrinsic reasons for learning about quality assurance and cost containment: to meet personal and professional demands for excellence, to respond to society's demand for accountability, to increase physicians' satisfaction in their work, and to improve the health and satisfaction of patients to whom care is provided. However, the transition from implicit concern with quality and cost to explicit, systematic programs and techniques that quantify and measure levels of quality and utilization of resources can be understood only in the context of the change in reimbursement for care that accompanied the changes in the way the health care system was organized and care delivered. To place the field of quality assurance in proper perspective, the reader needs to understand the historical roots of health care reimbursement, which will eventually force legislation requiring quality assurance systems as a matter of urgent national policy.

Shift to Third-Party Reimbursement. From time immemorial, medical care, like most professional services, was viewed as a private transaction between physician and patient. This does not mean that there were no codes or regulations governing the delivery of care or the fees charged. Indeed, there is evidence that some such codes were established by the profession and others by governments. (As early as 2000 B.C., the Mesopotamian Code of Hammurabi contained laws dealing with medical practice, fees, and costs. In the ninth century, Rhazes, an Islamic physician practicing in Spain, developed measures and criteria for differentiating trained physicians from pretenders.) For the most part, however, the physician's responsibility was to the individual patient, and fees for service were often set on the basis of ability to pay, with payment methods taking diverse forms, such as credit, payment in kind, and prepaid contracts. The exception to this system was, of course, service to the poor. In Europe, the churches undertook responsibility for providing care to the poor and paid physicians on an individual-case basis. In the American colonial period, town governments assumed this responsibility, and salaried "town physicians" cared for the sick poor (Roemer, 1945). As the colonial population grew, large towns built almshouses and established dispensaries where free consultation and treatment were provided. Attending physicians and apothecaries were paid an annual salary by a board of governors from money raised by charitable subscription. In the colonies, at least, this form of third-party payment was not without its limitations: The level of service was minimal, recipients of care were screened to ensure that they were among the "deserving poor," and access to care was firmly regulated, as were hours, salaries, and conduct of the attending physicians.

Federally organized health services originated in 1798 with the establishment of congressionally mandated compulsory health insurance for merchant seamen. A small sum was deducted from each sailor's wages to operate marine hospitals, but as these deductions failed to cover hospital costs, Congress was forced to make up the deficit (Terris, 1944). State governments assumed responsibility for the mentally ill; however, this service was provided for the same reason that prompted the creation of jails—to protect the social order. All the forms of publicly or privately funded medical care were characterized by a minimum level of care provided at minimal cost in institutions organized by respectable citizens for their social inferiors.

In contrast to the fee-for-service system based on the individual's ability to pay and the charitable free care to the poor or mentally ill, each of which left control of access and quality in the hands of the physicians or the funding source rather than within the power of the patients, certain forms of contract practice based on the concept of health insurance began to develop. Fraternal societies and mutual benefit associations, for example, provided sickness insurance to working men in the form of cash benefits. These "lodge practices," or medical prepayment plans, were popular forms of contract practice among many physicians glad to have assured income. By World War I, fraternal societies provided an estimated one half to two thirds of all health insurance in the United States. The remainder was supplied by trade unions and commercial insurance companies.

The recognition that access to medical care should be made available to the growing population incapable of making large out-of-pocket payments for care led to societal concern and government involvement in ensuring access to medical services. Germany and other European countries established compulsory health insurance systems in response to working-class pressures (Dawson, n.d.). In 1911 the British Parliament passed a National Insurance Act to provide health insurance to industrial workers. In the United States, several groups advocated forms of national insurance. The American Socialist Party called for sickness insurance in 1904. In 1912 Theodore Roosevelt's Progressive Party adopted a similar platform, and in the same year the American Association for Labor Legislation created a Committee on Social Insurance to prepare a model bill for introduction to state legislatures (Numbers, 1978). This bill proposed to provide income protection and complete medical care for manual laborers earning less than $100 a month, with premiums divided among workers, employers, and the state. Although the organized medical profession initially supported the legislation, commercial insurance companies violently opposed the bill, arguing that it would be disastrous for the medical profession and the quality of care. Organized labor was divided on the issue. Samuel Gompers, president of the American Federation of Labor, argued that the solution to the problem of access to medical care was higher wages, not compulsory insurance (Commission to Study Social Insurance and Unemployment, 1918). Eventually the medical profession was persuaded to oppose compulsory health insurance, and the prospect of any such legislation was dead by 1920.

The solution to the problem of access to care then took the forms of a series of bills to provide care for those in need and of an increase in the number of third-party insurers, particularly for hospital care. For example, the Sheppard-Towner Act (1921) provided federal funds to states for establishing prenatal care centers, conducting child health conferences, supporting visiting-nurse programs, and distributing informational literature. As a result of the Great Depression, hospitals were forced to find new methods of financing patient care and began to experiment with insurance schemes to cover hospital costs (Williams, 1932), which eventually became the Blue Cross plans. This prepaid hospital insurance provided an immediate solution to the problem of hospital financing but did not resolve the growing public demand for broader social security legislation. Consequently, the original draft of Franklin D. Roosevelt's Social Security Bill of 1934 included compulsory health insurance, a provision deleted from the Social Security Act of 1935.

In 1943 the Wagner-Murray-Dingle Bill again called for federally financed health insurance through extension of the Social

Security program, but this legislation too was defeated. Instead, as unions began organizing for group health insurance to meet rapidly rising medical costs, attention was redirected toward voluntary, or commercial, insurance. Inability to pay for medical care was no longer a problem restricted to the poor. Advances in medical technology resulting from the increased emphasis on medical research produced a growing number of medical specialists, research institutes, laboratories, and expensive equipment, thus increasing the costs of care. In addition, the expansion and modernization of hospital facilities, funded through the Hill-Burton program (1946), contributed to the continually increasing costs of providing modern hospital care. As a result, participation in group health insurance plans came to be considered a necessity, and enrollment in such plans was one of the major benefits available to employees, the employer assuming responsibility for negotiating the contract with the third-party payers. Thus, the traditional negotiation between the physician and patient with regard to fees and method of payment passed into the hands of these insurers of health care.

There still remained a sizable portion of the population for whom health insurance was not available: the elderly and the indigent. The Social Security Amendments of 1965 (P.L. 89–97) were intended to provide hospital and medical protection to these two groups. Through Medicare (Title XVIII), the federal government was to provide hospital and medical insurance protection to those sixty-five and older, to those under sixty-five receiving Social Security cash benefits or cash benefits from the railroad retirement program because of disability, and to certain chronic kidney disease patients. Under Medicaid (Title XIX), the federal government was to provide joint funding with state governments for medical care to the needy. With the enactment of this law, the federal government became one of the largest third-party payers for medical services. Not surprisingly, it became one of the first to experience the impact of the rising costs of care.

Effect of Third-Party Payment on Quality Assurance/Cost Containment Legislation. Nearly 25 million people became eligible for coverage under P.L. 89–97, increasing demand for health services throughout the country. The proportion of the GNP allocated to health care rose accordingly even though utilization review for

Medicare recipients had been included in the 1965 legislation and was extended to Medicaid programs by the 1967 Social Security Amendments (P.L. 90–248). Public expenditures (federal and state) for personal health care had risen from $6,976,000 in 1964–1965 to $23,987,000 in 1971–1972 (Cooper and Rice, 1976), prompting further legislation intended to monitor both the costs and quality of care provided to the populations covered by these programs.

The rapidly escalating expenditures associated with publicly funded programs such as Medicare (Title XVIII) and Medicaid (Title XIX) had, by the early seventies, provided sufficient impetus to a cost-minded Congress to secure the passage of Senator Wallace Bennett's Social Security Amendments of 1972, thus creating the Professional Standards Review Organizations (PSROs). Originally, the PSRO review was to cover care provided in institutions such as short-stay hospitals, mental health institutions, and skilled nursing and intermediate care facilities that participated in Medicare, Medicaid, and Maternal Child Health programs. The three major review mechanisms used by PSRO were based on concurrent admission certification and continued term care review; medical care evaluation studies; and analysis of hospital, practitioner, and patient profiles.

Given the focus of the PSRO program and the need to begin quality and cost assessment almost at once, it is not surprising that the initial approaches to assessment relied heavily on available data—that is, the medical record. Among the first methods to be implemented widely was utilization review. This method involves screening claims forms or medical record abstracts against explicit empirical criteria (average "practice" performance) and is intended to determine the appropriateness of hospital admissions, length of stay, and amount of ancillary services used. For cases noncompliant with the criteria, a follow-up implicit review of the record was to be conducted by a physician. PSRO programs have since placed more emphasis on the establishment of institutional and provider profiles, the improvement of Medical Care Evaluation Studies (MCEs), and more targeted review. Though initially quality assurance activity was focused on short-stay hospitals, currently steps are being taken to develop guidelines for review of both long-term and ambulatory care. The extension of PSRO activities beyond institutional care to ambulatory care and the broadening of the approach to quality assurance review indicate that the original legislation mandating quality assurance will soon affect all levels of health care delivery.

Recently the Office of Professional Standards Review Organizations (OPSRO), following the precedent established by the Joint Commission on Accreditation of Hospitals, announced that it will implement a new strategy to augment, if not replace, traditional chart audits of previous Medical Care Evaluation Studies. This approach, the quality of patient care study (QPC), will emphasize problem identification, data gathering and peer analysis, intervention for problem resolution, follow-up to assure improvement of the problem, and reporting and documentation of the study process and outcome. This approach will apply the principles developed in this text.

Undoubtedly the need to comply with federal regulations is the least satisfactory rationale for motivating the health care provider to learn about quality assurance and cost containment. It falls far short of the more intrinsic values of improving individual patient care and living up to the standards set by the profession. It is also less appealing than the arguments based on social justice. However, recent legislation on quality assurance and cost containment cannot be ignored. Future physicians, at some time in their careers, if not immediately, will need to know the origins of PSRO, the mechanisms for review, and the purpose of peer review. Furthermore, implicit quality assessment will be replaced by systematic programs of measuring and improving both the quality of care (effectiveness) and the resources used to provide that care (efficiency). Consequently, it is incumbent on every physician to learn how to conduct such a systematic quality assurance effort.

Evolution of the Private-Sector Mandate for Quality Assurance. In addition to the quality assurance activities resulting from new legislation, a number of developments in the organization of health care service extended utilization review to the private sector. For example, in the 1940s a group of physicians in California formed the San Joaquin Medical Foundation in order to provide some practice competition to the Kaiser-Permanente prepaid plans that were developing in that state. Subsequently, a number of large, county- or statewide medical care foundations (MCFs) similar to the San Joaquin model were formed. Although these MCFs were not themselves Health Maintenance Organizations (HMOs) in the strict sense, many of them sponsored a type of prepaid practice—namely, Independent Practice Associations (IPAs)—in order to compete with local HMOs. To remain competitive with the HMOs, the medical care foundations had to monitor carefully the utilization of health services (particularly inpatient services) among the physicians participating in the IPAs. In other words, these foundations initiated a form of utilization review very similar to utilization review prescribed later in the Bennett Amendments. Not surprisingly, as local PSROs were being established, many of the medical care foundations found themselves in the position of becoming the local or statewide PSRO. In many areas, utilization review, which these foundations had been practicing in the private sector, was extended to Medicare and Medicaid patients as part of the PSRO program.

As private industry grew increasingly concerned with the rising costs of health care, in part because of the effect on the cost of benefit packages offered to employees, many large companies became interested in the work of the medical care foundations in the area of utilization review. In 1977 the American Association of Professional Standards Review Organizations joined with the American Association of Foundations of Medical Care to form a nonprofit organization, Peer Review Network, Incorporated (PRN). Recently PRN has negotiated with large companies and labor groups and with their numerous health insurance carriers to provide organized utilization and peer review of all services offered employees through the various health insurance plans. Industry's interest in controlling health resource expenditures and its willingness to participate in programs to review utilization of these resources indicate that quality assurance activities may well extend more fully into the private sector.

Summary

This chapter has provided a brief overview of the rationales—professional, personal, and public—for participating in quality assurance activities. It has also defined quality assurance in such a way as to include assessment and improvement of both the effectiveness (quality) and efficiency (resource utilization) with which care is delivered. The following portions of this text explain the basic concepts that must be understood in order to conduct systematic quality assurance programs and illustrate how these concepts are applied in an actual practice setting. For those interested in pursuing the topic in greater depth, a series of data sources is provided in the appendixes to the text. Although it is difficult to capture the complexities of and changes in a field of study that is still evolving, as quality assurance is, the content of this volume can provide the reader with a basic understanding of the field and serve as a foundation for future study and research.

The Knowledge Base for Quality Assurance and Cost Containment

In a systematic approach to assessment and improvement of care, the first and most critical step is to identify topics and assign priorities for the quality assurance study or project. Many components of health care delivery could be monitored and evaluated on a routine, continuous basis: provider performance, condition of health care facilities, administrative procedures, clinical interventions, patient satisfaction, laboratory accuracy, and the like. However, because quality assurance efforts are limited by available resources, personnel, and time, the most effective approach to use in a systematic assessment of quality and cost is to focus on a known or suspected problem. Problems of inappropriate care and utilization can be identified in several ways. For example, utilization review conducted by Professional Standards Review Organizations (PSROs) identifies inappropriate hospital admissions and length of stay, as does the practitioner profiling used by the Professional Activity Study (PAS) of the Commission on Professional and Hospital Activities and the PSRO programs. Reports and findings of

13

various hospital committees, such as tissue review, blood utilization review, antibiotic usage review, and infection control committees, contain information that points to problems of poor quality or overutilization. Even routine sampling of the individual physician's medical record could reveal several areas where problems of cost or quality exist. So, too, would comparison of a hospital's performance with national or regional data serve to identify problem areas in the hospital, particularly with regard to length of stay and treatment modalities. Or one could use the formal group technique described later in this text, the nominal group process, to select and prioritize problems. Whatever the approach used, it is essential to focus the assessment effort on a known or suspected problem.

To apply this problem-oriented approach to assessing and improving the effectiveness and efficiency of care, one must understand certain basic concepts. The following portion of this chapter and Chapter Three explain these concepts, thus responding to the second question addressed in this text—What does one need to know to perform quality assurance studies? The specific types of information needed for conducting studies are drawn from several disciplines, including epidemiology, health economics, and behavioral and organizational psychology, and require knowledge of

- The range of health problems brought to the medical profession by society.
- The importance of these health problems to society as determined by the frequency of occurrence and associated health loss and economic costs.
- The efficacy and safety of available interventions as demonstrated under ideal conditions of care.
- Current effectiveness and efficiency with which these problems are being managed under usual conditions of care.
- The potential for achieving health care improvement by applying available methods for correcting the identified deficiencies.

This chapter and the next show how this information constitutes the basic concepts to be understood and applied in conducting a quality assurance study. Before discussing these essential

concepts, however, we will explain briefly the way health problems
are used as the organizing framework for quality assurance.

Health Problems: The Organizing Framework for
Quality Assurance Study

Although there are many components of health care that
could provide a focus for quality assurance efforts, the approach
described in this text uses health problems, the most fundamental
component of health care delivery, as the organizing framework
for the study because they are central to the delivery of care as well
as to quality assurance studies. For example, in the management of
a patient, the specific health problem is the focus of diagnosis and
therapy because

- It is because of symptoms of a health problem, or a desire to
  avoid them, that patients present for care.
- It is on the basis of the types of suspected health problem that
  providers decide on a particular diagnosic strategy.
- The nature of the health problem determines the therapeutic
  or preventive intervention used.
- The type of health problem, together with its complexity and
  severity, influences the cost of managing the problem.
- It is on the basis of health problem categories that health status
  is projected—that is, untreated to establish seriousness and
  treated to establish prognosis.

In conducting a quality assurance study, specific health
problems are used as the organizing framework for the reasons just
listed as well as because

- The content of medical practice in a given setting is organized
  according to specific presenting problems or diagnostic
  categories.
- National and regional data on frequency and costs of care are
  classified according to diagnosis of health problems or
  symptoms.
- Determinations of the efficacy of health care interventions are

made on the basis of their effect on specific health problems.

- Effectiveness and efficiency are measured in terms of the outcomes or processes of care applied to specific health problems in a given setting.
- Improvement potential is determined by assessing to what degree the health problem can be improved if deficient care is remedied.

To assess and improve the effectiveness and efficiency of diagnosis and treatment of health problems, it is necessary to have information on (1) patient reasons for contacting physicians and (2) diagnostic categories developed by providers. It is possible to arrive at an assessment of diagnostic effectiveness by comparing patient reasons for contacting physicians with the diagnoses arrived at by the providers on the basis of the symptoms, physical exam and history, and lab test results. The National Ambulatory Medical Care Survey provides statistical data that permit classification of health problems according to patient reasons for visit. This information is divided into three major categories: nonsymptom, common symptoms, and less common symptoms. Within the major catogories, the survey defines subcategories in which patients report symptoms according to the body system affected (see Table 2.1). If the quality assurance team were to try to discern whether false negative diagnoses (missed diagnoses) had been made for a particular health problem—for example, patients presenting symptoms suggesting acute myocardial infarction, such as acute chest pain, who were diagnosed as having a more innocuous health problem, such as pleurisy—it would need to assess the records of all patients having acute chest pain as the original reason for visit. Unfortunately, at present, patient complaint coding is not usually included on medical records, and hence it is difficult to assess diagnostic quality by any of the current forms of chart audit. However, it is recommended that in the future this type of health problem information be coded and cross-indexed to enable quality assurance personnel to assess diagnostic accuracy for patients with common presenting complaints.

Assurance of the effectiveness and efficiency of therapeutic judgment for specific health problems is somewhat easier because

Table 2.1. Common Patient Reasons for Ambulatory Care Visit (Illustrative Components of Leading Categories).

Nonsymptom

Well patient
Physical examination, insurance examination, "checkup," well-patient services, examination related to normal pregnancy and infancy

Nearly well patient
Asymptomatic follow-up of previous illness (medical, surgical aftercare)

Common Symptoms

Eye, ear, nose, and throat complaints
Infections and sequelae:
Sore throat, "cold," earache, sinus trouble, inflamed eye, chills, fever, cough, "flu"
Allergy
Impaired vision or hearing

Visceral problems
Chest pain, shortness of breath, "blood pressure"
Heartburn, gas, abdominal pain, vomiting, diarrhea
Menstrual cramps, intermenstrual bleeding, discharge
Urinary burning or frequency

Musculoskeletal problems
Pain, swelling, injury of head, neck, back, upper and lower limbs

Skin problems
"Acne," pimples, warts, allergy, minor wounds and lacerations

Emotional and vague general complaints
Anxiety, restlessness, depression, fatigue, "tired blood," loneliness, sexual problems

Less Common Symptoms

All other

---

data do exist on health problems categorized by diagnosis and appropriate treatment. By comparing the timing, quantity, modality, and type of treatment prescribed for a particular diagnosis against treatment criteria for that particular health problem, it is possible to assess the quality of the therapeutic judgment. In fact, this is the approach used in conducting medical audits (that is, assessment of medical care by using process data from medical records), and it enables quality assurance personnel to detect inappropriate or insufficient therapeutic care, assuming the diagnosis is valid. As mentioned earlier, however, the medical record does not enable quality assurance personnel to arrive at a thorough assessment of diagnostic quality. More significantly, the medical record does not provide information on the outcomes of care that require special follow-up observations.

Despite the shortcomings of the current methods of assessment that depend on recorded chart data, it is still expedient for quality assurance personnel to understand health problem categories and related data in planning health care assessment. Accordingly, in Appendix A of this text, resources that provide necessary information according to diagnostic and patient complaint categories are identified and their use in quality assurance studies explained.

Determinants of Health Problem Importance

Using health problems as the organizing framework for quality assurance is a practical and feasible way of acquiring information on health problem importance, a factor that must be taken into account in selecting and assigning priorities to topics for quality assurance study. Health problem importance concerns the cost to society of health problems themselves. It is determined by examining (1) the frequency with which certain health problems occur in a given population; (2) the amount of health loss attached to these problems; and (3) the economic costs associated with both health loss and the care provided to prevent, diagnose, and treat them. This portion of the chapter will define each of these determinants of importance and explain their implications for quality assurance study. Appendix A also provides sources of national and regional data on health problem importance.

Frequency. Frequency is the measure of the number of times a particular health problem occurs in a given population. Epidemiologists refer to this measure of health problem occurrence as morbidity and quantify it in terms of incidence and prevalence rates. Those attempting to measure health loss or economic costs of health problems in a given population automatically incorporate frequency rates in their calculations. For example, costs of care for hypertension in a local health maintenance organization (HMO) would be quantified by multiplying the cost of care per person by the number of persons involved.

For quality assurance purposes, it is necessary to know the frequency rates of health problems in the population of the setting under study in order to select a topic that meets patient sampling requirements and affects a sizable portion of the population. Otherwise, a problem may be selected for study that is so rare that it would require several years to accumulate a representative sample on which to base an assessment of physician performance. Or a study topic may be selected that involves considerable disability per person but affects relatively few people in that particular setting. The more prevalent health problems can yield the required sample size within a reasonable time.

One method of accurately estimating the frequency of a health problem is to conduct a direct sampling of patients in the practice setting where the quality assurance study is being performed. However, this method is costly and requires appropriate sampling and survey methods to yield valid results. An alternative approach to determining frequency is to identify local existing data compilations, available for most short-stay hospitals, or to consult national data and to extrapolate from these to the local setting.

Health Loss. Health loss encompasses a range of factors associated with health problems, including health risk, impairment, disability, mortality, and the social disruption that occurs in families or communities because of these factors. To conduct an assessment that includes an examination of health outcomes of care, it is necessary to have valid data on the mortality and disability resulting from particular health problems if untreated (natural history data) and on the degree of mortality and disability that can still be expected even when ideal care is provided. Knowledge of the expected type and extent of health loss associated with particular health problems enables quality assurance personnel to select topics that warrant study because of the potential for a considerable reduction in health loss if deficient care is improved. It also allows them to develop meaningful standards with which to judge the effectiveness of care and to select or design appropriate instruments for measuring the health outcomes of care. For example, if normal pregnancies (which are frequently seen in community hospitals) are to be the subject of the quality assessment study because of a suspected care problem, data on the expected population mortality or disability associated with this condition will allow those conducting the assessment to develop outcome criteria by which to recognize the presence and extent of excessive or preventable complications, avoidable degrees of pain and suffering, and unnecessary health risks. Similar information on expected health loss associated with myocardial infarction will assist quality assurance personnel in estimating the presence and extent of preventable losses of longevity and years of productive major life activity as well as avoidable suffering.

Economic Costs. Three types of economic costs are associated with a health problem: (1) the amount of direct care expenditures utilized to manage it—that is, treatment costs, (2) costs of iatrogenic disease, and (3) the earnings loss and opportunity costs associated with the problem.

Treatment costs refer to the relative value of the resources expended in the management of specific health problems. They include charges for services, value of time of personnel, and cost of equipment, supplies, and facilities used in diagnosis, therapy, rehabilitation, and long-term care. Often this type of economic cost is called the tangible, direct costs associated with a health problem. Quality assurance personnel need data on this type of cost in selecting topics for study, as this is one indicator of the importance of the health problem to society. Utilization review as conducted by the Professional Standards Review Organizations (PSROs) and the Commission on Professional and Hospital Activities (CPHA) has generated both national and local data on length of stay and utilization of service, thus providing one type of data on treatment costs categorized by diagnosis. The more recently developed case-mix methods (Fetter, Thompson, and Mills, 1976; Fetter and others, 1977, 1980; Mills and others, 1976; Thompson, Fetter, and Mross, 1973; Young, Swinkola, and Hutton, 1980) supply actual or estimated costs of treating specific health problems according to the complexity or severity of cases rather than according to number of hospital beds, ratios of residents to beds, or average days of hospitalization. Additional sources of data on this type of direct treatment costs are provided in Appendix A.

Costs of iatrogenic illness are also important to the quality assurance team as an indicator of health problem importance. Certain health problems carry a high risk of producing patient dissatisfaction with care or engendering unrealistic expectations for care outcomes. The costs of such problems should also be included in the quality assurance team's consideration of importance, as they often involve a high risk of avoidable malpractice suits, which increase the economic costs of care. One quality assurance technique, generic screening, has been developed to identify specific care outcomes that carry a high risk of legal action, such as internal bleeding in patients recovering from surgery or generalized sepsis in recently discharged hospital patients that results in emergency admission to the hospital and severe disability in patients receiving care for a fracture (Mills, 1977).

Earnings loss, productivity loss, and lost opportunity costs are the most difficult type of economic costs to quantify. To calculate productivity loss resulting from morbidity or mortality, it is necessary to take into account both the amount of productive time lost and the money value assigned to the lost output. Estimates of earnings loss resulting from premature mortality rather than from morbidity include in their calculations such factors as the increase in dollar value that would have occurred had the earnings been invested at the prevailing interest rate. Although risks are involved in adopting this "human capital" approach, which means valuing people as though they were machines and using productivity to measure the value of a life (Acton, 1976), it does provide one indication of what health problems are important to society. Hence, these indirect but tangible costs of health problems or disease (like the intangible costs of pain, suffering, and social dysfunction) should be taken into consideration when selecting and giving priority to health problems that warrant a quality assurance study.

Although it is relatively easy to understand why the three determinants of health problem importance—frequency, health loss, and economic costs—must be used in selecting topics for quality assurance study, it is extremely difficult to determine the value

	Health Loss	Economic Cost ($)
Illness-Related	**A** Disability and mortality encompassed by natural history of a health problem, plus intangible costs of pain, suffering, and social dysfunction	**C** Productivity loss and opportunity costs of illness (indirect costs)
Health-Care-Related	**B** Disability and mortality associated with professional management, plus intangible costs of pain, suffering, and social dysfunction	**D** Dollar costs of health care (direct costs)

Each cell implies population data that incorporate the factor of health problem frequency.

Figure 2.1. Establishing Health Problem Importance:
A Medical Framework.

attached to particular health problems on the basis of these determinants. Most health care practitioners are accustomed to establishing health problem priorities on the basis of health loss, giving lower priority to the other determinants of importance. Hence, if physicians were asked to assign priorities to illness-related and medical-care-related costs, they would undoubtedly rank them as shown in Figure 2.1.

The first indicator of importance to the physician would be that represented in Cell A—the risk, disability, or mortality produced by the illness itself. Next in importance would be Cell B, the related health loss produced by health care independent of the illness, or iatrogenic impairment (both preventable and nonpreventable). Cell C, the costs associated with the medical care of the

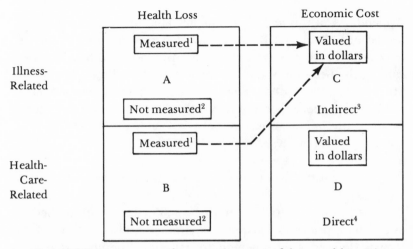

1. Quantifiable as time units (for example, years) of decreased longevity or added disability
2. Sometimes quantified as psychosocial cost of pain and suffering and other subjective factors
3. Quantified as productivity loss to society
4. Quantified as dollar costs/resources devoted to health care

Figure 2.2. Quantifying Health Problem Importance:
An Economic Framework.

given health problem (including preventive, diagnostic, therapeutic, rehabilitative, and long-term aftercare), would be ranked third by the physician in determining importance. Cell D, the earnings and productivity losses and lost opportunities associated with illness, would rank last.

Figure 2.2 represents an economic framework that might be used in determining health problem importance. Economists attempting to attach a dollar value to these same components in the health care field would develop a different order of priority (Pliskin and Taylor, 1977; Bunker, Barnes, and Mosteller, 1977). The direct costs of health problem management and the indirect costs of earnings loss due to mortality and morbidity would be used as the first two priorities for determining importance. (Sources of data that provide specific dollar estimates of these are presented in

Appendix A of this text.) The tangible and intangible costs represented in Cells A and B would have less priority for economists.
However, there are several different approaches to measuring or
valuing the health loss and economic cost of health problems (see
Hu and Sandifer, 1981). Such efforts are important for quality
assurance purposes because they help the quality assurance team
estimate the importance to society of health problems and then
select topics for study.

Efficacy of Health Care Interventions

A third concept that must be understood and applied in
establishing priorities for quality assurance study is efficacy. Efficacy is defined as the benefit to a defined population that is
achieved by health care interventions under ideal conditions of use.
Establishing evidence of efficacy usually requires the conduct of
clinical research studies in which a particular health care intervention, such as a preventive, screening, diagnostic, or therapeutic
management procedure, is applied to a particular health problem
in a defined population to determine the benefits of care. In conducting such studies to estimate efficacy, researchers carefully control the variables that affect the delivery of care in order to show
that the benefits achieved are directly related to the intervention,
not to some extraneous factor. They measure the results of the
interventions at a specific point in time, thus reaching conclusions
about the immediate outcomes of care (those occurring minutes or
days after the intervention), the intermediate outcomes (those occurring weeks or months later), and long-term outcomes (those
occurring years later). The types of outcomes they measure may be
those that affect patient health (for example, improved longevity,
reduction in disability) or those that affect the economic status or
degree of satisfaction experienced by either the patient or the physician. Appendix B presents sources of national data on efficacy.
    It is no surprise to most physicians that many of the inter-
ventions they use in caring for patients are of uncertain efficacy.
Many, if not most, interventions have not been studied systemati-
cally to determine and document their efficacy, nor is there a systematic procedure for identifying interventions that should be

studied. In fact, once interventions have become a part of health care practice because of customary use for particular health problems (for example, tonsillectomies and adenoidectomies for children to prevent recurring sore throats), it is extremely difficult to conduct the type of controlled study that is required to determine efficacy.

Those involved in performing quality assurance studies do not conduct clinical research studies to determine whether the interventions being used for care of the health problem under study are efficacious. Rather, their task is to find evidence that the intervention is efficacious, including evidence of the optimum benefit that can be expected from that intervention. Such evidence can be obtained by conducting a literature search or a direct review of recent clinical studies. The information gained in this search for documentation of efficacy serves several purposes. First, identification of the degree of expected benefit from an intervention under ideal conditions of use provides a standard against which to measure how effective the intervention is in the actual practice setting under study. Second, verification that a particular intervention is efficacious for the health problem under study can eliminate the possibility that the unsatisfactory outcomes are due to the use of an inappropriate intervention; conversely, if the search shows the intervention to be of doubtful efficacy, it may indicate that use of the intervention itself should become a quality assurance study topic. Finally, since documented evidence of efficacy includes information on characteristics of the patient population for which the intervention is effective, such evidence makes it possible to assess whether the intervention is being used on appropriate subjects in the study setting.

Characteristics of Efficacy Studies. In reading reports of efficacy studies for particular interventions, quality assurance personnel must note four things: the type of medical condition for which the intervention was applied, the specific condition of use, the characteristics of the population studied, and the benefits achieved.

The *medical problem* may be a disease, a symptom, a syndrome, or some other type of health problem for which the intervention was tested. Since some interventions are used for a variety of problems, it is important that the efficacy report specify which

LIBRARY
College of St. Francis
JOLIET, ILL.

102669

disease or condition was the subject of the efficacy study. For example, hysterectomies are used for treatment of premalignant states and localized cancer, for descent or prolapse of the uterus, for obstetric catastrophes, and as a prophylactic measure to prevent later cancer or pregnancy (Office of Technology Assessment, 1978). If hysterectomies are the subject of the efficacy report, the condition for which they were shown to be efficacious must be specified (for example, localized cancers). It cannot be assumed on the basis of such a report that hysterectomies are equally efficacious for the other conditions; it would be necessary to find reports that documented their effect on these other conditions. In addition, if the study shows that the surgery produced a certain benefit at one stage in the illness, one cannot conclude that it would produce the same type of benefit at another stage. For example, a total hysterectomy may be lifesaving for a Stage I cervical carcinoma but only palliative for Stage IV of the same problem.

Conditions of use include the timing, quantity, circumstances, and modality with which the intervention was applied, whereas *population characteristics* include the age, sex, and disease stage of the patients. If an intervention has been determined to be efficacious for a particular patient population, one can assume only that it will be efficacious for patients with similar characteristics. For example, in the Veterans Administration study of antihypertensive agents, the study population comprised men under 65 years of age with diastolic blood pressure above 105 mm Hg (Veterans Administration Cooperative Study Group on Antihypertensive Agents, 1970). The study did not include females, nor did the initial report indicate that patients with diastolic blood pressure in the range of 90 to 105 mm Hg had been evaluated. On the basis of this study, then, one could not assume that the antihypertensive agents would be efficacious in females or in those whose blood pressure was between 90 and 105 mm Hg.

The *type of benefit* may vary according to the type of intervention studied. Therapeutic interventions may produce benefits related to mortality and morbidity, but they may also have positive effects on longevity, palliation, and psychosocial functioning. Documented improvement of outcomes in any of these areas may be considered a benefit of the therapeutic intervention. Reports of efficacy of diagnostic interventions, in contrast, may define benefits in entirely different terms—for example, reliable performance, accuracy, or diagnostic impact.

Efficacy Study Designs.

1. *Diagnostic interventions and validation designs.* The technical accuracy of diagnostic tests used to confirm the presence or absence of disease is determined by a validation design (Figure 2.3). This type of study compares the results of the diagnostic test with those obtained from an existing procedure accepted as a clearly more valid indicator of disease—for example, coronary angiography for coronary disease compared with autopsy. A perfect test administered to fifty diseased and fifty well persons will produce fifty true positives (with disease), fifty true negatives (without the disease), and no false positives or false negatives. There are no perfect tests however. Tests vary in their sensitivity, or how well they detect the disease; in their specificity, or how much they avoid false diagnosis of the disease; in predictive value, or how often positive tests truly indicate that the patient has the disease; and in efficiency, or how often positive or negative results are truly positive or negative. All these characteristics must be evaluated to determine the accuracy of a diagnostic test. They are measured as follows:

$$\text{Sensitivity} = \frac{\text{true positives}}{\text{true positives and false negatives}}$$

The percentage of positives when patients have the disease

$$\text{Specificity} = \frac{\text{true negatives}}{\text{true negatives and false positives}}$$

The percentage of negatives when patients are free of the disease

$$\begin{array}{c}\text{Predictive value}\\ \text{of a positive}\\ \text{result}\end{array} = \frac{\text{true positives}}{\text{true positives and false positives}}$$

The percentage of all positives that are true positives

$$\text{Efficiency} = \frac{\text{true positives and true negatives}}{\begin{array}{c}\text{true positives and false positives and}\\ \text{false negatives and true negatives}\end{array}}$$

The percentage of all results that are true results

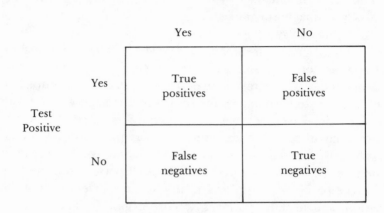

Figure 2.3. Validation Design Used to Determine the Diagnostic
Value of a Test.

Galen and Gambino (1975) provide an excellent explanation and illustration of these concepts.

2. *Therapeutic interventions and clinical trials.* The efficacy of therapeutic interventions is determined by the benefit to the patient, usually in terms of improved health outcomes. To determine whether the health outcome is the effect of the treatment and not of some other cause, controlled clinical trials (Figure 2.4) are used. In these trials the benefit of the treatment under study is compared with that of a placebo or an alternative treatment in terms of alleviation of symptoms, control of disease progression, increased length of survival, decreased morbidity, or cure. Among the types of trial used to assess therapeutic efficacy are the following:

- *Trial:* The simultaneous comparison of two or more treatments, one of which may be a placebo, to determine the relative benefit of the treatments.
- *Controlled trial:* An experimental method in which subjects are assigned, according to predetermined rules, either to an experimental group, which receives the intervention, or to a control group, which receives a standard treatment or placebo.
- *Randomized, controlled trial:* Subjects in a controlled trial are randomly assigned to experimental and control groups.

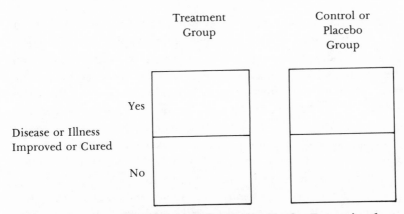

Figure 2.4. A Controlled Clinical Trial Design Used to Determine the Therapeutic Value of a Preventive, Curative, Rehabilitative, or Management Procedure.

- *Double-blind, randomized, controlled trial:* A randomized, controlled trial in which both subjects and clinical evaluators are unaware who receives and who does not receive treatment.
- *Sequential trial:* A trial whose conduct at any stage depends on the results so far obtained; usually the results influence only the number of observations made.

The therapeutic benefit depends on the objective of the intervention. For example, use of decongestant antihistamine combination drugs is intended to provide palliation of rhinitis, whereas lung resection for carcinoma is intended to cure this condition. It would be appropriate to assess the therapeutic efficacy of a drug such as that used to relieve rhinitis by a double-blind, randomized clinical trial, whereas the efficacy of a surgical intervention is more often assessed by means of a randomized controlled trial. The surgery in this case may be compared with no treatment or, more likely, another treatment, such as radiation therapy.

In addition to noting assessment of the efficacy of the therapy, one must also take note of reported evidence of its safety, which is determined in relation to the degree of risk associated with the intervention. Risks include adverse reactions, side effects, expected reactions, and idiosyncratic reactions. Because many interventions carry risks, it is important to decide what level of risk is acceptable. This is often determined by the severity of the medical problem, the characteristics of the population, or the conditions of use. For example, certain cancer chemotherapies, though efficacious as treatment, may produce bone marrow suppression. Given the severity of the disease, this may be considered an acceptable risk, virtually a side effect or an expected reaction; hence the intervention would be considered safe. However, if bone marrow suppression resulted from an anti-inflammatory drug used in treating acute tendonitis, a disease of much less severity, the intervention would be considered unsafe, as it produced an adverse reaction more severe than the condition being treated.

3. *Preventive interventions and case-control designs.* Preventive interventions are used to reduce risk attributable to a habit, life activity, or health care intervention. A reported study to estimate the efficacy of a preventive intervention must document the relationship between the activity or behavior and risk. The extent of risk associated with various behaviors has been studied extensively by epidemiologists and others. The study designs used to establish risk vary but generally are similar to the case-control design (Figure 2.5). The case-control design is used to determine the relative risk of illness, disease, or death in persons with a characteristic hypothesized to be detrimental to health, compared with those with a lower level of the characteristic or those without it. It may be used in prospective studies (to follow subjects forward over time while they are exposed to various levels of the health-impairing behavior) and in retrospective studies (to examine the effect of past exposures on present health status). Retrospective studies using the case-control design have provided estimates of the risk of carcinoma of the uterus associated with use of conjugated estrogens for menopausal symptoms, of death and disease associated with cigarette smoking, and of general thrombosis associated with use of oral contraceptives.

Once it has been established that risk is attributable to certain behaviors, habits, or health care interventions, it is necessary to note evidence of the efficacy of the preventive interventions intended to reduce risk. The ability of an intervention to reduce risk is the major measure of efficacy for preventive medicine. Study designs used to determine the efficacy of preventive measures are similar to clinical trials used for evaluating the efficacy of therapeu-

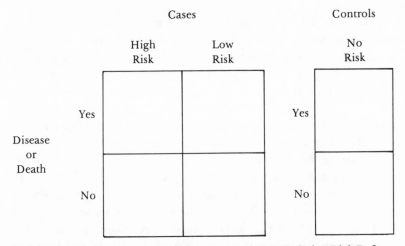

Figure 2.5. Case-Control Design Used to Document Relative Risk Before Disease Onset.

tic interventions. Because it is difficult to assess the effect of risk reduction on health outcomes, however, reduction in the purportedly noxious behavior is sometimes used as a measure of the efficacy of the preventive intervention. The following terms are associated with studies of preventive interventions:

- *Relative risk.* Rate of disease in a group exposed to the risk divided by the rate of disease in a nonexposed group.
- *Attributable risk.* Rate of disease in an exposed group that can be attributed to the exposure. Assuming the courses of diseases other than the one under examination had equal effect on the exposed and nonexposed groups, the rate of disease among nonexposed persons is subtracted from the rate among those exposed.
- *Cohort studies.* The group or groups of persons to be studied are defined in terms of characteristics appearing before the detection of the disease under study and observed over a period of time to determine the frequency of the disease among them.
- *Cross-sectional studies.* Characteristics being compared are present in the cases and controls at the time of the study.
- *Retrospective studies.* Characteristics being compared are sought

by data collection regarding past events (using medical records, patient and/or physician interviews, and the like).

• *Prospective studies.* Characteristics being compared are planned for future data collection (using direct observation or other, indirect methods).

References useful in further understanding these concepts include Lilienfeld (1976) and MacMahon and Pugh (1970).

In conducting the search for documented research evidence on efficacy, the quality assurance team needs to be familiar with the processes described above to assess the credibility of the studies it reviews. The design of the study, the precise nature of the results, and the authority of the authors must all be taken into consideration when the team is evaluating the studies. Gifford and Feinstein (1969) have provided an excellent illustration of how to review such studies critically.

The basic rules that should be followed by quality assurance teams conducting such studies may be summarized as follows:

• Search the literature.
• Examine the scope and design of the reported studies.
• Obtain information from national or local experts or peers.
• Evaluate the usefulness of identified sources.
• Use the information for developing the quality assurance plan.

In order to describe the results of a search, it is useful to record the result in terms of the amount and quality of the evidence identified. This involves describing the intervention and its relation to the problem for which it is used, the outcomes studied, and the population of concern. The evidence from the review is examined to see whether efficacy is manifest or not manifest. Efficacy of a procedure or intervention is said to be manifest when efficacy has been established in medical settings and is obvious to the observer, as in the case of cast applications for forearm fractures (Office of Technology Assessment, 1978). If efficacy is not manifest, one then notes whether the evidence has been studied or not studied. If studied, the evidence is described according to its location on two continua—sparse versus plentiful and conflicting versus concordant. If not studied, its status as under study, not under study, or

Health Care Intervention: _____

Problem: _____

Outcomes: _____

Population: _____

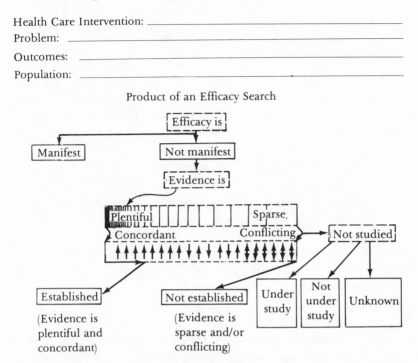

Product of an Efficacy Search

Note: Cochrane (1972) and the Office of Technology Assessment (1978) are two readable texts on the subject of efficacy.

Figure 2.6. Example of a Record for Documenting the Results of an Efficacy Search: Classification of Efficacy in Relation to the State of the Medical Literature.

unknown is stated. Then substantive statements about the efficacy of the intervention can be offered. Figure 2.6 illustrates one way of recording results of a search to document efficacy of a particular intervention.

Effectiveness and Efficiency of Health Care

Knowledge of the efficacy of health care interventions is a precondition for measuring the actual effectiveness of the health care provided and the efficiency with which it is delivered. It is these two characteristics of health care—effectiveness and efficiency—that are measured in order to plan and implement actions intended to achieve improvement in care. This section of the chapter will define effectiveness and efficiency, distinguish these concepts from efficacy, and discuss ways they are measured. Sources of data on effectiveness and efficiency can be found in Appendix C.

Defining the Terms. In the health care literature, the terms *efficacy, effectiveness,* and *efficiency* are frequently used as if the same definition applied to all. What was called efficiency in the early 1900s by Codman (1916) and later by Querido (1963) is now called effectiveness; Cochrane (1972) uses the terms *effectiveness* and *efficiency* interchangeably. In health service research these terms have very distinct meanings. As mentioned earlier in this chapter, *efficacy* refers to the benefit achieved by health care provided to a defined population under ideal conditions of use. *Effectiveness* is the benefit achieved by health care provided under usual conditions of care. *Efficiency* is the extent to which health care effectively achieves its inherent efficacy with a minimal expenditure of resources.

To understand the differences among these three concepts, consider an analogy. Passenger trains are designed to transport people from one location to another. They can achieve this desired outcome when tracks have been properly laid, skilled personnel run the trains, and passengers adhere to fixed schedules. When these last-mentioned conditions are present (ideal conditions of use), passenger trains have been shown to be an efficacious transportation intervention. The effectiveness of this method of transportation under usual conditions of use may be less than its demonstrated efficacy. For example, the condition of the roadbeds may be poor and the personnel less skilled than required; untoward events may occur, such as derailments; or passengers may fail to arrive at the scheduled departure time or to reboard the train after a stopover. The efficiency with which this intervention operates—that is, with minimum cost and within a reasonable expenditure of resources—varies from one country to another. For example, "featherbedding," wherein unions force railroad companies to assign firemen to trains even though they no longer have a function, illustrates how passenger trains may incur unnecessary costs that decrease efficiency but have little influence on effectiveness.

Similar occurrences in health care delivery under usual conditions can influence the effectiveness of an otherwise efficacious intervention (for example, patient noncompliance, inadequate professional performance, untimely or inappropriate levels of care) or the efficiency with which it is delivered (for example, unnecessary laboratory tests or operative procedures, inappropriate use of emergency rooms, or prolonged stay in hospitals or long-term care facilities). To determine the degree of effectiveness or efficiency with which care is provided and to improve that care when it is found to be deficient, quality assurance studies must be conducted. The Institute of Medicine (1974) expresses the relationship of effectiveness and efficiency to quality assurance as follows: "The primary goal of a quality assurance system should be to make health care more effective in bettering the health status and satisfaction of a population, within the resources which the society and individuals have chosen to spend for that care." In this statement, effectiveness is defined in terms of the health and satisfaction outcomes of health care; quality assurance is seen as a means of improving these outcomes and increasing the benefits of care. By implying that these outcomes should be achieved within the limits of the resources available for care, the statement indicates that a review of the costs associated with health care is an essential part of quality assurance as well.

General Approaches to Evaluating Effectiveness and Efficiency. The state of the art of effectiveness and efficiency assessment is in flux, and new methods are still being developed. Several techniques exist, however, that should be understood, the two most commonly used general approaches being medical audit and utilization review. Medical audit, which can be based on either implicit or explicit criteria, uses process data from medical records to assess effectiveness and efficiency of care. In an audit based on implicit criteria, physicians review the entire patient record and judge whether the process of care is acceptable. In an audit using explicit criteria, nonphysicians review the records against predetermined criteria developed by physicians to ascertain whether care has met the predetermined criteria. In utilization review, claims forms or medical record abstracts are reviewed to determine appropriateness of admissions, length of stay, and ancillary services. The records or claims forms are screened against explicit empirical criteria, such as the "average performance in practice." Follow-up implicit review is conducted by physicians for those cases that do not comply with the criteria.

Two other general approaches, interview and direct observa-

tion, rely on the judgment of outside observers. Interview has not been as widely used as medical audit, but when employed as an assessment method, it usually focuses on patients. Direct observation assesses the process of care as it actually occurs or retrospectively through use of videotapes or films.

Current Assessment Techniques.

1. *Those using predetermined criteria to assess care processes.* Several techniques that rely on predetermined criteria of the process of care have been developed to assess effectiveness and efficiency. For example, *bi-cycle* is a two-step assessment process that involves (1) selection of clinical problems having high priority for study on the basis of the amount of disability caused and (2) assessment of how well actual practice complies with predetermined performance criteria for these high-priority problems (Brown and Fleisher, 1971). Discrepancy between criteria and actual performance indicates physicians' need for continuing medical education. After physicians complete their continuing medical education, their patients' records are reassessed to see whether care has improved. *Educational patient care audit* is a retrospective assessment using the medical record to determine compliance with predetermined criteria (California Medical Association/California Hospital Association, 1975). This method has two unique features: (1) practitioners being evaluated must ratify the predetermined criteria, and (2) they must set a "threshold for action," or a minimum percentage of charts that must meet the predetermined criteria in order for care to be considered acceptable. If the threshold is exceeded, then corrective action must be taken. *Concurrent quality assurance,* developed by Private Initiative in PSRO, is a technique that examines specific diagnoses against three categories of predetermined criteria developed by a panel of experts: diagnostic criteria, documentation criteria (that is, required information on the medical record, such as morbidity, predisposing factors, severity, and complications), and treatment criteria (that is, efficacious and contraindicated treatment). In this technique, immediate outcome data are posted prominently in the charts of participating patients. The actual assessment of adherence to criteria is done concurrently by nonphysician reviewers (Sanazaro and Worth, 1978).

2. *Those using predetermined criteria for other purposes.* Predetermined criteria are also used in three other techniques to assess

(1) the quality of clinical decision making (criteria mapping), (2) the presence of potentially compensable events due to medical management (generic screening), and (3) the presence of certain tracer conditions that indicate a problem of care (tracers). *Criteria mapping* uses a decision tree that identifies the numerous sequential decisions to be made for a given clinical problem and provides several alternatives for each step of the decision process (Kaplan and Greenfield, 1978). Predetermined criteria of performance are used to assess compliance at each step, or node, in the decision process. *Generic screening* uses twenty generic criteria that could be applied across all diagnoses and clinical problems to identify such events as hospital-incurred trauma, adverse drug reactions, readmission to the hospital, and mortality to determine whether these events could lead to malpractice suits (Mills, 1977). This technique originated with the California Medical Insurance Feasibility Study. *Tracers* (Kessner, Kalk, and Singer, 1973) evaluate process and outcome for a single specific common health problem on the assumption (as yet unproved) that it will provide an assessment of the entire care delivered. The tracer health problem selected must conform to six criteria: It must have functional impact; be well defined diagnostically; be of high prevalence; be amenable to influence by medical care; be characterized by a clear understanding of prevention, diagnosis, treatment, and rehabilitation; and include an understanding of effects of nonmedical factors. To assess the quality of care for "tracer" health problems, criteria for the minimally acceptable level of care must be applied. These criteria should focus on practical forms of care rather than sophisticated technology and be based on the population at large rather than individuals.

    3.   *Outcome-based assessment techniques.* Certain other assessment techniques focus on the outcomes of care. *Problem Status Index/Outcome* (PSI), used to measure ambulatory care outcomes, involves sending questionnaires to patients at a predetermined time after contact with a health care provider for a specific clinical problem (Mushlin, 1974; Mushlin and Appel, 1978, 1980). Frequency and severity of symptoms as well as limitation of activity are assessed and compared with the expected results of acceptable health care for that condition. The observed outcomes are also correlated with process information contained in the medical record. *Staging* (Gonnella and others, 1977) assesses outcomes of care

by classifying patients according to three levels of severity of the health problem on entrance into the health care system—(1) no complications or minimal severity, (2) local complications or moderate severity, and (3) systemic complications or maximal severity—and measuring the change in stage over time. Effectiveness and efficiency of care are determined by the proportion of a group of patients with a given diagnosis who are at each of the three stages of severity, compared with accepted standards. The underlying assumption for this method is that high severity on entrance may indicate inadequate accessibility or inappropriate management before entrance. Levels of severity for comparable populations can be used as standards against which to compare the distribution of severity among the patient population under study.

4. *Assessment techniques focusing on problem identification.* Problem identification may also be the focus of the assessment technique. *Health Accounting* is a problem-oriented approach that uses a combination of assessment techniques, depending on the problem—for example, medical record review, observation, or patient follow-up survey. This approach involves incremental learning of practical methods for estimating and documenting both the costs and benefits of health care. Ultimately, use of acceptable tools of health status assessment of patient populations (health accounting) is given as much administrative emphasis as financial accounting currently receives. Three generic categories of benefits are measured: health, economic, and societal. This approach emphasizes measurement of outcomes in a cyclic assessment-improvement strategy (Williamson, 1978; Williamson, Alexander, and Miller, 1967; Williamson and others, 1975). The *Comprehensive Quality Assurance System,* developed by the Northern California Kaiser-Permanente Medical Centers, begins with review of a small sample of charts by two practitioners to identify problems in patient care. The results of this screening review are presented to the quality assurance committee, which selects the most significant problems for further assessment and sets standards for the selected problem areas. Charts are then reviewed to determine compliance with the standards set, and noncompliant charts are subject to implicit review by a physician to ascertain whether there is a problem of unacceptable quality. Where true problems of quality are iden-

tified, corrective action is taken and reassessment follows (Rubin and Kellogg, 1977). *Quality Assurance Monitor* was developed by the Commission on Professional and Hospital Activities as a service available to hospitals. By examining hospitalwide, departmentwide, and diagnosis-specific or surgery-specific groups on a continuing basis, it is possible to identify priority problem areas that require further detailed study. Each monitored hospital receives a "priority for investigation" listing that indicates where the hospital's performance is substandard compared with other hospitals of the same type (Lowe, 1977a, 1977b).

The comprehensive approach to the conduct of quality assurance described in this text recognizes that the quality assurance team may use some or all of the foregoing techniques in assessing and improving the effectiveness and efficiency of care. The critical elements of the process advocated here are that the study be health-problem-oriented and that priorities be assigned on the basis of the importance of the health problems (that is, their frequency and associated health loss and economic costs).

Most of the current methods rely on information that can be recorded in the health care record or gathered by a silent observer. They result in an assessment of providers' knowledge or of their motor skills and information-gathering ability. However, they do not provide a method for assessing providers' analytical thought processes, clinical judgment, or decision-making skill, all of which are critical to provision of quality care. Cognizant of this gap in current assessment techniques, researchers are now investigating the application of decision-analysis methods to quality assurance.

Summary

This chapter has identified concepts that must be understood before undertaking a quality assurance study to assess and improve the effectiveness and efficiency of care in a particular setting.

Specific health problems are the most feasible and appropriate focus for structuring quality assurance planning. By examining the health problem content in a given practice setting, it is possible to discern which health problems occur most often and to ascertain which of these problems carry the heaviest risk of health loss or consume the largest portion of the health care dollar. In other words, using health problems as the organizing framework for quality assurance permits selection of topics that warrant study by virtue of their frequency as well as their associated health loss and economic costs.

Furthermore, quality assurance personnel (and health care providers) must be able to ascertain whether there are interventions capable of producing benefits to the population afflicted with a given health problem. Knowledge of the expected benefit to be achieved by applying a particular health care intervention to a given population under ideal conditions of use is derived from documented reports of efficacy of health care interventions. Understanding what efficacy means and how clinical research studies are conducted to determine efficacy enables quality assurance personnel to evaluate the efficacy reports for particular interventions and to develop realistic standards against which to compare the actual health care delivered in the setting under study.

Assessment of the actual delivery of care for a particular health problem in the study setting is accomplished by measuring the effectiveness and efficiency of that care to determine where and to what degree there is potential for improvement. As defined in this chapter, effectiveness relates to the benefits actually being achieved through use of the health care interventions in current community practice. Several techniques are used to measure effectiveness (for example, health accounting, staging, and concurrent quality assurance, to name but a few). Efficiency is defined in terms of the resources used to achieve the benefits of care. The main method currently in use to measure efficiency is utilization review. Understanding of the concepts of effectiveness and efficiency is crucial to quality assurance, since the measure of effectiveness and efficiency is what allows the quality assurance team to determine the improvement potential, the fifth basic concept of quality assurance, which is discussed in the following chapter.

Identifying the Potential for Improvement in Health Care

ౠౠౠౠౠౠౠౠౠౠౠౠౠౠౠౠౠౠౠౠౠ

One additional concept, improvement potential, must be understood in order to conduct effective quality assurance studies. Improvement potential involves identification of (1) the benefit that could be achieved if deficient care were to be improved and (2) currently existing methodologies that could be applied to achieve the desired improvement. Although there are no regularly published data as such on achieving improvement, a number of publications provide useful information on this concept. These publications are listed in Appendix D.

By comparing the results of the effectiveness and efficiency measurements of the care being provided in the given setting against the benefits that could have been achieved, it is possible to identify an area that has potential for improvement in care. However, before deciding to focus the improvement plan on this area, it

41

is important to ascertain whether methods are available for bringing about the desired changes in provider or patient behavior and attitudes that will produce the achievable benefits. In other words, it is necessary to determine that a "treatment" exists to correct the problem with the care provided and to select from among the existing "treatments" one that corresponds to the type of problem identified.

For this aspect of the quality assurance study, one turns to the fields of adult education, industrial engineering, systems analysis, and organizational development, which rely heavily on the behavioral sciences, for developing methods for changing individuals, organizations, and systems. Application of these methodologies requires an understanding of how professionals act and define themselves, how various components or subgroups within an organization interact, and how changes in individuals and organizations actually occur.

In planning for improvement in health care, it is important to recognize the three main interacting components of any health care encounter: the patient, the practitioner, and the organizational structure. Taken together, these interacting components may be viewed as a system to which the concepts of and techniques for change from the aforementioned disciplines can be applied. At any point in time, the patient's health status is influenced not only by the process of care (whether preventive or curative) provided by the practitioner but also by the patient's own attitudes and behaviors and by such organizational variables as equipment, personnel, policies, and procedures.

When problems in quality of care, such as less than optimal achievable patient health status, are identified, change activities must take into account not only the role of the practitioner but also those of the patient and the organization. However, attention to problem identification and quantification alone, without equal attention to the skills needed to *solve* such problems, is destined to produce frustration and to reduce the impact of any quality assurance efforts to improve health care (Williamson, Alexander, and Miller, 1967; Jessee, 1977b). This section of the text, then, will examine the characteristics of each component of the health care encounter that affects health status and improvement planning and will suggest practical approaches to use in achieving improvement.

The Process of Planned Change

The process of achieving improvement through quality assurance is analogous to that of planned change, which, as defined by Schein (1972), involves learning new ideas and concepts, new attitudes and skills, and new patterns of behavior. Planned change can be divided into three stages: (1) unfreezing, or unlearning of present ways of doing things; (2) developing new beliefs, values, and behavior patterns; and (3) refreezing, or stabilizing and integrating new beliefs, values, and behavior patterns. It usually involves both a change agent and a process through which change can occur.

The change agent, whether internal or external to the system, must have such competencies as conceptual diagnostic knowledge, familiarity with the theories and methods of organizational change, knowledge of sources of help, and awareness of the ethical and evaluative functions of the change agent's role (Bennis, 1969). In other words, the change agent must be able to identify the problem and the individuals or subsystems affected by the problem, assess their readiness to change, communicate and share information with the members of the subsystem or system, and provide necessary and appropriate education (Beckhard, 1969).

The change process involves creating motivation to change, acquiring new information to assist in developing new attitudes or responses, and integrating the new responses or attitudes into the behavioral patterns of the individual or the functioning of the system. In quality assurance activities, the quality assurance team, composed of members of the health care institution who assume a new or additional role within the institution, can be considered a change agent. This team must have many of the competencies of the individual change agent, including ability to assess the care being provided and to diagnose the problems affecting health, satisfaction, or economic outcomes; familiarity with information resources that can clarify the nature of the problem; knowledge of methods and approaches to correct the problem; and ability to involve providers, patients, and institutional administrators in seeking or implementing solutions.

Bennis (1969) has identified the steps to be taken by the change agent: identifying the appropriate point of entry into the organization, diagnosing the interdependencies within the system, involving those who will be affected by the change in goal setting and planning, obtaining voluntary commitment of participants, and selecting approaches to achieving change that are congruent with the goals and values of the institution or organization. Translating these steps into quality assurance means that the team must be able to identify the clinical department, clinical subgroup, or patient population to whom the improvement actions are to be directed; enlist the cooperation of key staff in setting standards or developing criteria; obtain support of department chiefs or chief administrators as well as of those who will be affected by the improvement activities; and adopt procedures that are compatible with the goal of improving patient care.

Improving Patient Compliance

Since patient behavior and attitudes are important determinants of health care outcomes, particularly in compliance with therapeutic or preventive regimens, improvement planners should understand some of the forces that shape this behavior and apply techniques that are successful in modifying it. Becker and Maiman (1975), in their "health beliefs" model, postulate that patient preventive health behavior is controlled by (1) the individual's perceived susceptibility to health problems and perception of their severity; (2) the individual's assessment of the "benefits" of the proposed health action as opposed to the "costs," whether economic, physical, or psychological; and (3) "cues to action," either internal or external, that interact with the predisposing patient perceptions to produce the health action. In addition, Becker and Maiman point out that patient compliance is shaped by (1) predisposing factors, such as motivation, value of illness threat reduction, and probability that compliant behavior will reduce the perceived threat; (2) modifying factors, such as age, sex, race, attitudes about health care, access, and economic status; and (3) enabling factors, such as prior experience with illness or treatment and social pressures.

There is a rather extensive body of research on techniques for modifying patient behavior by altering patient perceptions and beliefs. For example, increasing the patient's perceived (subjective) level of vulnerability has been shown to be effective in increasing compliance with practitioner recommendations in such areas as cancer screening (Flach, 1960; Kegeles, 1969; Fink, Shapiro, and Lewison, 1968; Haefner and Kirscht, 1970), tuberculosis (Hochbaum, 1958), and heart disease (Haefner and Kirscht, 1970). Becker, Drachman, and Kirscht (1974) also have reported increased compliance with oral treatment regimens among mothers who believed their children to be susceptible to recurrence of otitis media. Similarly, patient estimates of the seriousness of an illness are consistently predictive of compliance with the prescribed medical regimen (Becker and Maiman, 1975). Since these techniques are based on theories of behavior modification, it is important that those planning to use them to achieve improved patient compliance recognize that it is essential to determine what patients value and to give these values priority over any institutional or social goal.

Other techniques to improve patient compliance rely on adult learning principles. Those involved in adult education note that learning takes place when the learner perceives a need to know something and that learning is more effective when the learner participates in planning the educational process and when the process is adapted to accommodate learners' individual differences and prior knowledge. For example, patient ownership of the medical record can improve patient self-sufficiency and physician/patient relationships (Bouchard and Tufo, 1977; Tufo and others, 1979). In a study to test the efficacy of joint goal setting by practitioners and patients, Starfield (1978) noted a higher level of concordance and better coordination of care than that achieved through traditional means of continuity. These and other studies on patient education, life-style modification, and patient self-care provide many suggestions for approaches to improving compliance and patient satisfaction. These sources are invaluable in planning approaches to achieve improvement.

Improving Provider Performance

Equally important in improving health care through quality assurance is the ability to effect change in the performance of health care providers. As with patients, a series of attitudes and characteristics are common to most professionals and must be recognized before an improvement action can be designed and implemented. As summarized by Schein (1972), characteristics of professionals include control of a specialized body of knowledge acquired by prolonged education and training, exercise of a high degree of autonomy in making judgments and decisions on behalf of clients, a detached, neutral attitude toward clients, cultivation of a relationship with clients based on mutual trust, a strong orientation toward service, and a position of power and status in the area of professional expertise.

Change agents must recognize these characteristics in selecting approaches to achieve improvement. For example, given the tendency of professionals to operate autonomously, it may be necessary for the quality assurance team to include techniques for promoting collaboration among health care providers, quality assurance personnel, and administrative staff in their improvement planning. One approach to fostering a sense of collaboration would be to involve the providers in setting standards or criteria for the quality assurance activity at the outset of the study. In this way, they would be better prepared for accepting the results of the initial assessment of the quality of care and for participating in the improvement actions. Similarly, recognition that professionals have a high degree of orientation toward service may mean that the improvement planner can appeal to providers' altruism to motivate them to change behavior, particularly if providers are convinced that better-quality patient care will result.

Some of the fundamental principles of human psychology and adult education applicable to patients are also useful in planning for improvement of provider performance—for example, the adult education principle that adults learn when they perceive a benefit to themselves in doing so (Knox, 1977) or the behavior modification approach, which identifies a reward system for persons in whom behavior change is desired.

One technique widely advocated as a tool for improving professional competence is continuing medical education (CME). During the past ten years, the frequency of requirements mandating specific hours of continuing medical education as a prerequisite for physician relicensure has risen dramatically. Yet there is little evidence that mandatory CME is associated with increased physician competence (Bertram and Brooks-Bertram, 1977; Jessee, 1977a), except in several isolated cases. For example, Ogilvie and Ruedy (1972) describe a significant improvement in the care of patients receiving digitalis preparations immediately after an intensive CME program on digitalis therapy at a Montreal hospital. Williamson, Alexander, and Miller, (1967) described a classic case in which knowledge-based continuing education programs failed to produce improved care in terms of response to unexpected laboratory test abnormalities, whereas subsequent education to change old habit patterns succeeded dramatically. Laxdal and others (1978) reported significant improvement in physician prescribing practices following an intensive, problem-based program of CME over a one-year period, whereas MacDonald (1975) has recently described the favorable impact of a "computer reminder" system, using algorithms to assure adequate evaluation and follow-up of outpatients under treatment for diabetes mellitus. Such approaches to modifying physicians' behavior are important tools to be incorporated into plans and activities for improving physician performance.

All these approaches to practitioner behavioral change assume that the individual is responsive to altruistic incentives or can be motivated to change by appeals to self-interest or self-improvement. However, it is also important to recognize that economic motives play a role in determining behavior and that these motives may conflict with altruistic goals. For this reason, it is appropriate to consider a variety of available economic sanctions that could be used in improving provider performance:

- Mandatory preadmission review of elective hospital admissions.
- Mandatory consultation or surgical assistance for certain diagnoses or procedures.
- Reduction, modification, or suspension of hospital privileges.
- Sanctions under the PSRO law, such as recoupment of Medicare/Medicaid payments, removal from participation in Medicare/Medicaid, or civil fines.
- Denial of insurance payment for inappropriate, unnecessary, or poor-quality services.
- Suspension or revocation of licensure.

Improving Organizational Functioning

Many of those involved in quality assurance activities acknowledge that a substantial proportion of the identified problems in patient care require improvements in the administration or structure of the health care institution. Effective planning to improve organizational functioning, and consequently patient care, can incorporate the theories and techniques for effecting change in individuals, and these theories can be supplemented by those derived from the relatively new fields of organizational psychology and systems analysis and from broad concepts of organization development. A thorough discussion of these theories, particularly as applied to health care service, would require a text in itself. However, it is useful for the purpose of this discussion to point out some characteristics of organizations to be considered when attempting to achieve improvement in organizational functioning and to explore techniques that bear further investigation.

Schein (1970) defines an organization as "the rational coordination of the activities of a number of people for the achievement of some common explicit purpose or goal, through division of labor and function, and through a hierarchy of authority and responsibility." Implied in this definition are characteristics of an organization that must be taken into account when attempting to change organizational functioning. For example, it is necessary to understand the individual diversity, the types of subgroups and subsystems, the interactions among subgroups, the interdependency of human and technological factors, and the levels of authority that constitute any given organization. Because of their complexity, organizations often seem resistant to change. This particularly applies to hospitals, as they are among the most complex organizations in any industry from the point of view of operating time, personnel, and levels of authority. Hospitals operate twenty-four hours a day, seven days a week. Hospital personnel range from the most highly skilled professionals to the unskilled, all with critical responsibilities for the success or failure of care. The organizational structure is such that medical and administrative staff function as "equals" with overlapping areas of responsibility, both answering to a board of trustees that may know little or nothing of the technical aspects of the institution's operation. Hospitals are described as having "diverse goals, diffuse authority, low task interdependence, [and] few performance measures" (Weisbord, 1976), all of which contribute to the difficulty of effecting organizational change.

Despite the problems associated with effecting change in hospitals, the relatively new field of organization development has been successfully applied in the hospital industry (see Drexler, Yenney, and Hohman, 1977a; Weisbord, 1974; Lawrence, Weisbord, and Charms, 1974). Furthermore, many of the concepts used in this approach (for example, Gestalt, transactional analysis, normative reeducation, interpersonal and group dynamics) are already known to the quality assurance "change agents," derived as they are from the behavioral sciences included in the medical school curriculum.

Conflict management is one aspect of organization development that can be particularly valuable to quality assurance change agents. Lawrence and Lorsch (1969) have written extensively on the relationship between an organization's ability to manage conflict situations constructively and its efficiency, productivity, and product quality. The most productive organizations are those in which managers (or change agents) are able to clearly *differentiate* the positions of the parties to a conflict and then proceed to *integrate* the various points of view into an acceptable compromise to which all parties can commit. Of the styles of conflict management described by Drexler, Yenney, and Hohman (1977b)—pantisocratic, autocratic, democratic, and laissez faire—the pantisocratic is the most productive. It fosters the cooperation, collaboration, and commitment that are essential to effective teamwork in that all personnel involved in the decision-making process have input and contribute to the final decision. Organizations using this style of conflict management are likely to have higher morale, lower turnover, less illness, and higher productivity than those using another dominant mode of conflict resolution. By advocating a style of conflict management that promotes such collaboration and cooperation among the members of a given institution, quality assurance change agents have a greater chance of success in improving organizational functioning.

Seven Suggestions for Promoting Change

To achieve the desired changes in provider performance, patient compliance, or institutional effectiveness, seven simple rules can be applied (R. E. Thompson, personal communication):

Be sure of the facts. Before a change action is initiated, change agents must be sure that their data are accurate and that they have complete information on the problem. Without this accurate and complete information, the credibility of the change agent can be compromised to such an extent that he or she becomes totally ineffective. For instance, a medical audit finding that weights are not recorded on infants seen in the emergency room for gastroenteritis clearly indicates the existence of a patient care problem. However, attempts to remedy the problem by providing physician or nurse education would not only fail but also be detrimental to the entire quality assurance program if the cause of the problem were found to be the lack of a baby scale in the emergency room!

Take appropriate action. In deciding what constitutes appropriate action, change agents should recall that attempts to change provider, patient, or organizational behavior may be perceived as an attack on self-worth and hence become a source of tension. Approaches that increase tension are more likely to stimulate rationalization and opposition to change than are approaches that make the point clearly but minimize the threat to the ego of the individual (or organization) concerned.

For instance, in a quality assurance study of treatment of

asthma in children where physicians failed to comply with the agreed-on criterion that arterial blood gases should be taken at least once for each patient, two strategies for changing provider behavior could be attempted. An autocratic approach would be to send a letter, signed by the medical audit chairman and marked "Personal and Confidential," to physicians who failed to comply with the standards set by the department of pediatrics. The letter would inform the provider that this was unacceptable practice, state that compliance would be expected in the future, notify the provider that his or her practice in this area would be monitored during the next six months, and warn him or her that failure to meet the criterion during that time would be grounds for modification of practice privileges. This approach is likely to produce hostility, defensiveness, and a conviction that "they" (that is, the medical audit committee) are wrong, resulting in no change in provider behavior. An alternative strategy, more in keeping with a pantisocratic approach to conflict management, would involve an informal meeting between the medical audit chairman and each noncomplying physician to allow the chairman to present the findings of the study with regard to the physician's behavior, to explain why the blood gases were considered important, and to elicit an opinion from the noncomplying physician on the ordering of blood gases to improve management of asthmatic children. In adopting this approach, the committee chairman might learn that as a result of many years of treating such children the physician had developed a personal set of criteria that took into consideration the trauma to the patient and the expense of blood gases. This approach is likely to lead to a productive discussion of substantive patient care issues and to modification in the behavior of both the noncomplying physicians and the rest of the staff.

State the problem specifically. If the problem is not clearly understood, it is difficult for any individual or organization to respond positively to the change initiative. Failure to be specific and direct in identifying the problem can produce anxiety and resistance. Therefore, a direct statement of the problem, including its severity and the potential consequences of leaving it unresolved, is essential.

State the desired solution. Not only must the problem statement be specific, but the solution desired by the change agent should also be clearly stated. Too often, individuals or organizational units are told only, "You have a problem—fix it." A specific possible solution, in operational or behavioral terms, is more likely to produce the type of change envisioned by the change agent. For this reason, it is important to give careful consideration to alternative solutions and to be able to suggest the desired alternatives before initiating the change interaction.

Be prepared to answer the "So what?" question. Before initiating the change activity, careful thought must be given to what the consequences would be if the individual (or unit) that is to be the focus of the change effort continued with the present behavior. If the present behavior has no adverse impact on patient care, risk, or resource utilization, it is probably not worth the cost (in both human and economic terms) to attempt the change. For instance, if one physician routinely uses intramuscular penicillin for otitis media, while the majority of his colleagues use oral amoxicillin, the change agent must consider carefully the consequences of permitting the first physician to remain "out of compliance" with the behavior of his peers. If no adverse consequences (patient outcomes, exposure to risk of injury, or unacceptably high cost) are evident, then it may *not* be appropriate to seek change. Medical practice and health care delivery are sufficiently diverse to allow for a number of acceptable approaches to patient management. Attempts to force rigid compliance with a single approach are likely to meet with failure unless one mode of care has clear advantages over another.

Don't force the issue. Excessive zeal in trying to make the point that change is required may produce the same type of resistance that results from an authoritarian change strategy. The harder the change agent pushes to make the point or to elicit an admission of responsibility, the harder the object of the change activity will resist. For this reason, the change agent must control the normal human tendency to force the issue. Stating the problem clearly and describing the desired change fully imply belief in the theory of "rational man"—that when informed of a problem and its solution, a "rational man" will take action to correct the problem. People are much more likely to conclude that change is in their best interests if allowed to consider the issue, weigh the advantages and disadvantages of change, and reach their own conclusion concerning the desired behavior. Forcing the issue often results in a further determination on the part of the individual or the organization *not* to change, as a demonstration of power, and it is counterproductive to the objective of improving care.

Use concurrent monitoring to ensure that new behavior is maintained. Behavior within organizations (such as hospitals) is often determined as much by convenience, administrative procedures, and habit as by the knowledge and skills of people within the organization. To ensure that the improved behavior is maintained, therefore, it is important to establish mechanisms for concurrent monitoring of the performance of the individual or organizational unit. This monitoring also serves to protect patients against adverse consequences if the undesirable behavior should persist. For example, if failure to record daily weights on patients with congestive heart failure is found to be the patient care problem, and appropriate action is initiated, the review coordinator might engage in concurrent monitoring of this aspect of nursing performance until it is evident that the problem has been corrected and a new behavior integrated.

Summary

This chapter has shown that knowledge of theories and techniques to encourage change in both individuals and organizations is as critical to quality assurance as is knowledge of the more clinical concepts of frequency, health loss, economic costs, efficacy, effectiveness, and efficiency. The discussion of the theory and concept of planned change indicated that the most accurate diagnosis of the health care problem and the most valid assessment of factors contributing to that problem will not produce the desired improvement unless effective techniques for changing individual and organizational behavior can be applied. The body of knowledge and skills used in managing change is not unlike that of the highly specialized field of neuroendocrinology: Not all physicians need in-depth knowledge of the field, but an understanding of the rudiments is an important part of physician competence. Similarly, to be an effective physician and an effective member of the quality assurance team, one must be able to make a diagnosis of the organizational problem and know where and when to contact a subspecialist who can treat that problem if health care improvement is to be achieved.

To test your understanding of the concepts described in Chapters One and Two, a self-evaluation exercise follows. In addition, sources of data on each of the essential concepts have been provided in Appendixes A–D, organized according to the concepts to which they relate. Appendix E provides reports and studies of quality assurance activities, including cost/benefit analyses of these activities.

The next chapter will illustrate how quality assurance is actually conducted. A case study demonstrating the five stages of quality assurance will be used, and the conceptual material from this chapter will be integrated into the discussion of this five-stage approach.

Suggested Self-Evaluation Project

The following hypothetical case history describes how members of a cardiology department in a large university hospital might respond to a suspected problem in quality of care. This case illustrates many of the principles discussed in Chapters Two and Three. A series of questions is presented at the end of this case to allow you to evaluate how well you have understood these principles.

A cardiology fellow in the division of cardiology of a large university hospital, Dr. Al Weghsrite, had indirectly accused another fellow of mismanaging three coronary catheterization patients. Dr. Kathy Tursaton, the chief of the division, overheard his remarks and felt that they raised two serious questions that needed to be answered: (1) Is the diagnostic procedure being used for assessment of coronary artery stenosis accurate and consistent? (2) Are recommendations to perform coronary artery surgery or to treat medically consistent and valid? To obtain answers to these questions, Dr. Tursaton proposed that the complaining fellow design and conduct a study of all the division's patients receiving coronary artery catheterization to confirm or refute his impressions. When asked how he would know which arteriogram interpretations and operative assessments were "correct," Dr. Weghsrite stated that as some of the faculty members and fellows were substantially better than others in assessing the presence and degree of stenosis and in making considered operative recommendations, he would compare the better stenosis assessors and operative judges with those not in that group. Dr. Tursaton questioned whether a "better" group existed and, if such a group existed, doubted whether the individuals who were better stenosis assessors would also be the better operative judges and vice versa. However, she suggested that Dr. Weghsrite review the literature on the accuracy of coronary arteriography, giving particular attention to methods of stenosis assessment and the efficacy of coronary artery bypass surgery compared with medical treatment.

Dr. Weghsrite reviewed the literature but found very little on methods of stenosis assessment in relation to arteriogram accuracy. He presented his review to the division's research conference with a proposal (1) to identify anonymously, by secret ballot, the division's best stenosis assessors, (2) to identify in the same manner the division's best operative judges, and (3) to conduct two studies. The division's faculty and fellows accepted his proposal and identified one fellow, one full-time faculty member, and one part-time faculty member for each group. For the first study, ten otherwise operable patients were reviewed by each fellow and faculty member in the division. Results showed that at least two of the three best stenosis assessors (stenosis criterion group) agreed 90 percent of the time, whereas the other fellows and faculty members agreed with the majority opinion of the stenosis criterion group 60 percent of the time. An association between length of cardiology experience and agreement with the best stenosis assessors was noted: Faculty members and fellows with two or more years of experience agreed more often with the stenosis criterion group than those with less than two years' experience. The second study, separate reviews by each fellow and faculty member in the division of ten additional patients of varying operability, showed that the best operative judges (operative criterion group) agreed with one another 80 percent of the time. The rest of the division agreed with the majority opinion of the operative criterion group 75 percent of the time. However, the variability within the division was distinct and patterned; agreement among faculty members was considerably less than agreement among fellows.

Dr. Weghsrite had difficulty interpreting the results of these studies. Dr. Tursaton suggested that the findings on stenosis assessment corresponded to a training effect. Though surprised at the lack of "improvement" beyond two years of experience, she accepted the results as meaningful within the limits of the study and hypothesized that the findings on operative assessment corresponded to an ideological dispute. Moreover, three predominant views of the efficacy literature were represented within the division. The fellows tended to follow one view, which happened to correspond with that of the division chief and that of another nationally recognized, senior, full-time faculty member. The extent of agreement among fellows was attributed to the "coercive" influence of the training environment, and it was hypothesized that their agreement five years after the fellowship would be less.

These findings were presented to the division, which, after heated discussion over the course of several meetings, agreed to the following recommendations:

1. New fellows would be formally introduced to methods of stenosis assessment early in their fellowships.
2. The coronary artery cineangiograms for each patient of a fellow would be reviewed independently by two faculty members for estimates of degree of stenosis. If the two disagreed, a third faculty member would be asked to estimate stenosis.
3. The faculty members would conduct a year-long seminar series. During this series they would review with the invited principal investigators from each major coronary artery bypass efficacy study their views of the indications for the procedure. After the series, the faculty would attempt to develop consensus criteria for the operative indications. These would be used as the division's criteria. A monograph based on this process would be written, with grant funding of the entire activity.

A repeat study of stenosis assessment one year later showed that the net effect of the stenosis assessment effort had been to increase the rate at which agreement was achieved. Fellows now took six months to reach a level of agreement previously achieved in two years. In the initial study, significant stenoses had been overdiagnosed more often than underdiagnosed. In the follow-up study, overutilization and underutilization were roughly equivalent. As a result, proportionately fewer patients of fellows were being operated on at the time of the follow-up study than at the time of the initial study. The direct cost savings to patients was estimated to be $150,000.

A repeat study of operative assessment two years after the initial one showed that the net effect of the operative assessment effort had been to decrease the variation observed among the faculty. The monograph had been produced and provided a single standard for operative indications within the division. In addition, the division's seminars became more lively with each report of a new efficacy study. Although conformity to the single standard in practice was not required, defense of practice based on the division's indications was mandatory. The result was some increased conformity but even greater debate and faculty communication. It was estimated that 20 percent fewer operations were recommended for stable angina in the repeat study, whereas 40 percent more operations were recommended for other forms of angina (and for no angina). Although the net effect on costs was negligible, quality of care was felt to be more consistent, and faculty development resulting from the process was generally viewed as exciting.

Questions

1. There were two suspected problems in this hospital setting. One related to the intervention used to diagnose coronary artery stenosis, the other to the use of coronary artery bypass surgery as a therapeutic intervention for managing coronary catheterization patients.

   a. Show that, on the basis of the three determinants of health problem importance (frequency, health loss, and economic costs), these suspected problems would warrant study.

Suggested approach: Consult national data on common health problems seen in short-stay hospitals categorized by diagnosis to determine relative frequency (that is, prevalence and incidence) of health problems for which these interventions are used. Consult national data on health care expenditures to confirm the view that these interventions involve substantial direct costs (management of problem) and indirect costs (pain, suffering, lost opportunity, and earnings loss).

b. Were the two original questions asked by the chief of cardiology related to efficacy or effectiveness and efficiency of medical care? Substantiate your answer.

2.   What local data could be consulted to confirm the judgment that these problems are important and warrant a study?

3.   The suspected problems in this setting raise questions about the efficacy of both the diagnostic and therapeutic interventions used by the hospital staff in managing coronary patients. In searching the literature for documented evidence of the methods used to diagnose coronary artery stenosis, what type of study design would Dr. Weghsrite expect to find described in the reports? What characteristics would he look for in the reported study to determine whether the report results were valid? How would the accuracy of the diagnostic tests have been measured? In searching for evidence of efficacy of coronary artery bypass surgery, what type of study design would he expect to find reported in the literature?

4.   Dr. Weghsrite found very little documented evidence of the efficacy of methods of stenosis assessment in the literature. Consequently, he adopted another approach in order to estimate the accuracy and validity of the staff's stenosis assessment. What approach did he use, and is it an accepted method of arriving at standards by which to judge the effectiveness of care provided in a given setting?

5.   Several techniques are described in Chapter Two for conducting assessments of effectiveness and efficiency. The approach

used in this study to determine which therapeutic intervention was appropriate for coronary patients resembles some of these assessment techniques. In your judgment, which of the techniques are most like the one used in this study? Are there other techniques that could have been applied to the problem?

6. Select one assessment technique that you might have applied to this problem and describe how you would have proceeded to conduct the effectiveness/efficiency study in this case. (Reminder: The references provided in Chapter Two should be consulted to obtain a full description of the chosen technique.)

7. The improvement plan used in this case was targeted toward improving physician performance in the areas of stenosis assessment and operative assessment. What aspects of the improvement plan corresponded to the theories of planned change described in Chapter Three? How did the improvement action incorporate techniques suggested in this chapter for improving provider performance? What other steps might have been taken to plan and implement the improvement?

8. Evaluating the results of the improvement action is a critical final step in conducting a quality assurance study. What steps were taken to reassess the study? What evidence was reported that indicated that the improvement action had been successful? In your opinion, did the study prove that the improvement in stenosis and operative assessments was a direct effect of the improvement action? Why or why not?

A Five-Stage Approach to Quality Assurance and Cost Containment Projects

ꙮꙮꙮꙮꙮꙮꙮꙮꙮꙮꙮꙮꙮꙮꙮꙮꙮꙮꙮꙮꙮꙮꙮꙮ

Two of the questions that this book proposed to answer have been addressed in the preceding chapters. Chapter One showed how quality assurance and cost containment has become an integral part of current medical practice; Chapters Two and Three explained what types of information are required to conduct quality assurance studies. This chapter responds to the question of how to conduct these studies in an actual practice setting.

The Five Stages of a Quality Assurance Study

A comprehensive study to assess and improve the effectiveness and efficiency of care progresses through five stages:

- Stage I. Topic selection and prioritization (problem identification).
- Stage II. Initial assessment (problem verification).

60

- Stage III.   Definitive assessment/improvement planning (problem cause/resolution planning).
- Stage IV.   Implementation of improvement actions (problem resolution).
- Stage V.   Reassessment (problem resolution documentation).

This problem-oriented approach to quality assurance has recently become mandatory for hospitals to meet the requirements of the Joint Commission on Accreditation of Hospitals (JCAH) and the Professional Standards Review Organization (PSRO).

Stage I, topic selection and prioritization, is analogous to the first step of clinical management of a patient, which is to elicit the major problems in the initial work-up and assign priorities to them. To select topics for quality assurance study and assign priorities to these topics, the basic concepts discussed in the previous chapters must be brought into play. In other words, the quality assurance team examines the health care problems seen in the practice setting under study and makes its topic selection on the basis of:

- The importance of the health problems encompassed, as determined by their frequency and the magnitude of health loss and economic costs associated with them.
- The known efficacy and safety of available interventions to address these health problems under ideal conditions of use.
- The current effectiveness and efficiency of health care by which these problems are currently being managed under ordinary conditions of practice and the extent of improvement potential.
- The availability of known and effective methods for correcting identified deficiencies or achieving care improvement that is judged possible.

To establish problem priorities, it is necessary to have (1) professional personnel, preferably an intradisciplinary team, to make judgments; (2) input information, preferably available data or results of previous studies, from a variety of sources that suggests potential problem topics; and (3) a method of formulating problem hypotheses, preferably by structured group judgment, based on both the available data and professional experience in the given setting. The task of choosing the quality assurance team usually falls to the person charged with executive responsibility for the study. This person must assemble a representative team capable of developing a useful list of quality assurance topics. Ideally, the coordinator of quality assurance is a physician with interest and experience in the field who can select other staff members to participate in the priority-setting process. The particular mix of personnel most suited by interest and background to jointly develop a quality assurance topic list will probably differ in each institution. However, the persons selected must form a group that can provide a balanced overview of the institution's functions, especially in terms of effectiveness and efficiency of the care provided.

Experience has shown that a core group of knowledgeable and respected staff physicians is essential to provide (1) expertise on efficacy and safety of clinical interventions and (2) personal judgment of present levels of clinical performance in their institution. In addition, nurses, technicians, administrators, and front-desk personnel should be included to represent other functional areas of the institution. Their different perspectives and knowledge of such problems as the level of present personnel performance, workloads, interpersonal relations, and condition of equipment and facilities can prove as important as purely clinical knowledge in identifying areas of possible deficiency and in analyzing the probable benefits and costs of a recommended quality assurance project.

The nominal group technique developed by Delbecq at the University of Wisconsin School of Industrial Engineering (Delbecq, Van de Ven, and Gustafson, 1975) is one approach that seems well suited to priority setting. A modified version of this approach (Williamson, 1978) requires the priority team to meet for a two-to-three-hour session to identify and prioritize topics, using available data and literature.

Stage II, initial assessment, is similar to the process of taking a patient's history, completing a physical examination, and performing laboratory tests to obtain data needed to test the clinical hypotheses encompassed in the problem list from the initial work-up. For the quality assurance team, the intent at this point in the study is to test the hypothesis that there is a specific problem of care in the study setting. This function requires criterion measurements and assessment standards to confirm the suspected problem. The assessment methods selected for use at this stage will depend on the problem being studied.

Stage III, definitive assessment/improvement planning, is analogous to formulating the differential diagnosis in clinical practice to establish probable etiology and treatment considerations needed to develop a therapeutic plan. At this stage of the quality assurance project, the team examines additional data or conducts brief literature searches to determine the probable cause of the deficiency or problem confirmed during the initial assessment (Stage II), checks the hypothesis on which Stage II was based, and validates the data and assessment standards for the study. The purpose is to make a valid formulation of the problem and its probable cause so as to select or create a plan to improve care that is responsive to the nature of the problem. This stage is finished when the improvement plan is complete.

Stage IV, implementation of improvement actions, is much like taking therapeutic action in clinical practice—for example, providing prescriptions, conducting surgery, or providing patient education. In conducting the quality assurance study, the team implements the plan for improvement, taking into account characteristics of the local setting, providers, and patients. The plan of action will have been identified during Stage I and modified and made explicit during Stage III to ensure that it is an effective way of correcting the identified deficiency. As the improvement action is being carried out, the team will solicit feedback at certain intervals to determine whether further refinement or modification of the improvement action is required.

Stage V, reassessment, resembles the actions taken in clinical practice to assess the effectiveness of the therapy—for example, return visit or rechecking of laboratory results. The quality assurance tasks to be accomplished at this stage include repeating the initial assessment study to ascertain the extent of the improvement and establishing with certainty which aspects of the improvement actions were responsible for the improvement. If this reassessment shows that no improvement occurred, the team must test its original hypothesis, consider other causes for the deficiencies in care, consider other improvement actions, and develop and implement a new plan (that is, re-cycle through the five stages). If reassessment verifies that improvement has occurred, it is then necessary to establish evidence that this change was likely related to the quality assurance actions, not to an outside variable.

To illustrate how these stages are applied in actual practice, we next present a quality assurance case study, based partly on data and events of an actual study (Williamson and others, 1975).

Applying the Five-Stage Approach: Case Study

Stage I: Selecting a Topic and Setting Priorities. The first of the five major stages of a quality assurance/cost containment study is conducted to elicit the chief problems in quality and costs of health care in a specific area of the practice setting examined.

In a health maintenance organization (HMO), a prepaid multidisciplinary group clinic with 23,000 enrollees, the eleven-member quality assurance/cost containment priority team consisted of the executive director, medical director, director of nursing, medical records analyst, clinic manager, representatives of four clinical specialties, and two consumer representatives. This group considered a number of topics for review, including management of urinary tract infections in females, follow-up of abnormal laboratory findings in general, use of skull roentgenogram in minor head injury, management of otitis media in children, and hypertension control in adults.

In a meeting that used modified Delbecq techniques of nominal group process (Delbecq, Van de Ven, and Gustafson, 1975), the priority team reached a decision, by consensus, to investigate the HMO's management of hypertension control in adults aged 35–65. The subject was suggested through a systematic review of the literature and data from HMO clinic charts provided by two staff members, to be referred to as the "staff team," who, out of personal interest, had previously researched this topic.

1. *Assessing health problem importance.* Accepting the basic concept that a topic must be important in order to warrant study, the team proceeded to examine the frequency of this health prob-

lem and the magnitude of health loss and economic costs associated with it. To determine the importance of the topic in terms of frequency, an analysis of medical records was conducted. It revealed a diagnosis of hypertension in 2,188 of the 9,000 enrollees aged 35–65 (24.3 percent of the group at risk). Further analysis showed that 828 of 4,500 enrollees aged 35–50 (18.4 percent)and 1,360 of 4,500 enrollees aged 51–65 (30.2 percent) had hypertension diagnosed. By comparing this distribution pattern with national data, the staff team confirmed that prevalence of hypertension in the enrolled population was almost identical to the national norm.

The staff team also estimated the number of enrollees with mild hypertension (diastolic pressure 90–114 mm Hg) and more severe hypertension (diastolic pressure 115 mm Hg or more). The estimates were based on national statistics (that is, advance data from *Vital and Health Statistics,* prepared by the National Center for Health Statistics, 1976) indicating that the ratio of mild to severe hypertension in the general population is approximately 3:1. As a basis for calculations, then, the team made the following assumptions about the HMO's enrolled patients with hypertension:

Age	Total Number with Hypertension	Number with More Severe	Number with Mild
<50	828	208	620
>50	1,360	340	1,020
Total	2,188	548	1,640

The team conducted a brief literature review (Kannel, Wolf, and Dawker, 1978; Stamler and Epstein, 1972; American Heart Association, 1974). This review reinforced the team's conclusion that the incidence of strokes, coronary artery disease, cardiac failure, and renal impairment is likely to be higher in groups of patients with uncontrolled hypertension. The staff team then consulted data on the incidence of sequelae of hypertension (stroke, myocardial infarction, cardiac failure, renal impairment, and death), using studies on large populations of treatment with controls (Veterans Administration Cooperative Study Group on Antihypertensive Agents, 1967, 1970, 1972; Smith, 1977, 1979).

Applying VA study rates for severe hypertension in all age groups and on mild hypertension in those aged 50 and over, as well as Smith's data for mild hypertension for those under age 50, the team made calculations based on these rates and arrived at the following risk prediction for the HMO's enrolled hypertensives over the next five years *if none were treated:*

	< Age 50	*> Age 50*	*Total*
Stroke	54	300	354
Myocardial infarction	118	107	225
Cardiac failure	94	131	225
Renal impairment	37	79	116
Death	4	272	276

The team then calculated the probability of these sequelae if all patients were *completely controlled* over the next five years:

	< Age 50	*> Age 50*	*Total*
Stroke	0	78	78
Myocardial infarction	55	97	152
Cardiac failure	0	0	0
Renal impairment	4	12	16
Death	4	37	41

Given the *frequency* with which sequelae of hypertension occur in untreated and in treated groups, the team had thus defined one of the three determinants of the importance of this topic. It then set about to calculate the other two determinants, *economic costs* and *health loss*.

The staff team estimated that, for enrollees, the cost for an average hospitalization was $4,400 for stroke, $5,500 for myocardial infarction, $2,000 for congestive heart failure, and $5,000 for renal impairment (Acton, 1975). In making these calculations of direct treatment costs, the team considered only short-stay hospitalization costs—that is, those posing potential monetary losses to the HMO. It elected not to consider other treatment costs, such as those that would be incurred in extended care facilities or from home nursing. Nor did they consider patients' earnings or loss of opportunities or the economic impact of loss of life or disability on other members of the family. All these costs, of course, are quite important to the patient enrollees and to society in general.

A precise figure could not be assigned to the health loss associated with each of the potential sequelae to uncontrolled hypertension. However, it was obvious to the team that sequelae carried a high degree of disability, pain, and suffering, all sufficient to underscore the importance of this health problem.

2. *Assessing efficacy.* Having established the importance of the topic, the staff team then set out to investigate whether efficacious management practices existed that could assure, under optimal circumstances, that patients with hypertension could be controlled to the extent described above. They cited reports on the efficacy of (1) controlling hypertension and (2) reducing the sequelae of hypertension in both mild and severe cases through the use of oral antihypertension agents, such as hydrochlorothiazide, hydralazine, hydrochloride, reserpine, and rauwolfia serpentina (Veterans Administration Cooperative Study Group on Antihypertensive Agents, 1967, 1970, 1972; Smith, 1977, 1979). The optimal effect of these therapeutic interventions obviously depends on optimum patient compliance. Optimum patient compliance is likely to depend on appropriate patient and physician education. A literature review provided evidence of efficacious programs that could be applied to patient and physician education, thereby improving compliance (Inui, Yourtee, and Williamson, 1976).

3. *Determining effectiveness and efficiency.* Next, on the basis of discussion that reflected their personal experiences and a review of the experiences of others (Brook, Williams, and Rolph, 1978), the staff team concurred that it was likely that an unacceptably large portion of the HMO enrollees with diastolic hypertension was out of control and at risk of serious complications. They hypothesized, on the basis of combined group experience, that the effectiveness and efficiency of their present control programs were below acceptable levels. They also concluded that it would be a relatively simple matter to test this assumption by measuring blood pressures on a sample of enrollees known to have hypertension and by recording the degree of control.

It was estimated that two thirds of the enrolled hypertensives were under control. Assuming a 67 percent control rate, the probability of sequelae in five years would be as follows:

	< Age 50	> Age 50	Total
Stroke	18	144	162
Myocardial infarction	78	100	178
Cardiac failure	31	42	73
Renal impairment	16	38	54
Death	5	115	120

The team set, as an achievable goal, a 95 percent level of hypertension control. Assuming a 95 percent control rate, the probability of sequelae in five years would be as follows:

	< Age 50	> Age 50	Total
Stroke	2	78	80
Myocardial infarction	58	97	155
Cardiac failure	4	6	10
Renal impairment	5	14	19
Death	4	37	41

Applying the costs per hospitalization to the probability of sequelae at the 67 percent control rate, the team estimated costs to be as follows:

Sequela	No.	Cost/Hospitalization	Total
Stroke	162	$4,400	$ 712,800
Myocardial infarction	178	$5,500	$ 979,000
Cardiac failure	73	$2,000	$ 146,000
Renal impairment	54	$5,000	$ 270,000
			$2,107,800

Current costs: $421,560 per year

Applying the costs per hospitalization to the probability of sequelae at the 95 percent control rate, the team estimated costs would be:

Sequela	No.	Cost/Hospitalization	Total
Stroke	80	$4,400	$ 352,000
Myocardial infarction	155	$5,500	$ 852,500
Cardiac failure	10	$2,000	$ 20,000
Renal impairment	19	$5,000	$ 95,000
			$1,319,500

Achievable costs: $263,900 per year

Thus, over a five-year period, if control of hypertensive patients could be improved from the present estimated 67 percent level to 95 percent and maintained at that level, the staff team estimated that in a population of 2,188 aged 35–65 with mild to severe hypertension the following number of admissions could be averted:

Stroke	82
Myocardial infarction	23
Cardiac failure	63
Renal impairment	35

This would amount to a savings to the HMO of $788,300 over five years, or $157,660 per year.

4. *Identifying effective improvement actions.* Finally, the staff team envisioned several interventions (provider or patient education) that the HMO could use to correct the situation should a study confirm that, indeed, an unacceptable number of patients were out of control. In other words, by comparing the results of the present effectiveness study (those under control under current programs) against the known efficacy of certain effective education programs (Inui, Yourtee, and Williamson, 1976), the team could predict that it would demonstrate a precise, measurable improvement potential to which some known efficacious educational programs could be applied, thus justifying the study.

Discussion. The priority team chose this topic for study for several reasons. First, as the data compiled by the staff team showed, the health problem (hypertension) was important by reason of its frequency in the study setting, the amount of health loss it could engender in the population, and the economic costs that would be incurred by the HMO in providing treatment. By comparing the expenditures for acute care hospitalization alone (excluding long-term care, home nursing, and earnings loss) at the 67 percent and 95 percent control levels, the priority team accepted the estimate that the HMO stood to save an average of $157,660 per year. This savings would more than pay for the yearly cost of an effective education program. In addition, other treatment costs, earnings loss, and health loss (disability), which would be high for patients not under control, would be prevented.

Next, the priority team concluded that efficacious programs exist that improve patient compliance with efficacious oral medication, thereby reducing the potential for stroke, coronary heart disease, cardiac failure, and renal impairment. Futhermore, the priority team envisioned that a relatively simple study could be conducted to ascertain the current degree of effectiveness in controlling hypertensive enrollees.

Finally, the priority team had several interventions to use in improving control should the study in fact show a large improvement potential.

Thus, the priority team gave this topic highest priority primarily on the basis of evidence previously compiled by two staff members having a personal interest in this topic.

Stage II: Initial Assessment. In clinical management of an individual patient, the second step consists in verifying the existence of a health problem by history taking, physical examination, and laboratory testing in order to develop a differential diagnosis. In like manner, in Stage II of a quality assurance study it is necessary to verify the assumptions that a problem exists and that it is of sufficient importance to justify a study.

Up to this point the priority team's decision to study control of hypertensive patients had been based on an assumption that this was a serious problem for the HMO. Now the team members set out to verify, through data collection, whether the problem was actually as serious as they assumed it was. The priority-setting team appointed a study team led by the two staff members who had developed data on this topic and also including a clinic nurse, the assistant administrator, and a physician extender.

1. *Methods.* To make an initial assessment of the extent of the perceived problem, the study team investigated a one-month consecutive sample of 248 walk-in patients having essential hypertension. These were patients who had at least one previously recorded diastolic pressure reading greater than 110 mm Hg. On each visit during the study, three independent blood pressure readings were taken with the patient in a resting state. It was agreed that if these three readings averaged less than 100 mm Hg, the diastolic blood pressure was under control. The study team set a standard of 5 percent as the maximum acceptable noncontrol rate. In other words, if the average of the three readings was above 100 mm Hg in more than 5 percent of the sample of hypertensive patients, more definitive study of this problem would be indicated.

2. *Results.* The study revealed that 36 percent of the 248-patient sample was out of control. In Stage I of the quality assurance process, the team had estimated that one third, or 33 percent, were out of control; therefore, this study verified the initial assumption that a problem existed. The binomial goodness-of-fit test showed that 36 percent represented a statistically significant deviation from the 5 percent standard set by the team.

When the calculation formulas used in Stage I were applied to the 63 percent control rate revealed by the sample study, it was estimated that there existed a risk, over five years, of the following sequelae and costs:

Sequela	No.	Cost/Hospitalization	Total
Stroke	170	$4,400	$ 748,000
Coronary heart disease	186	5,500	1,023,000
Cardiac failure	78	2,000	156,000
Renal impairment	56	5,000	280,000
			$2,207,000

If the goal of 95 percent control were achieved (see estimates for Stage I at 95 percent control rate), the difference between this and the 63 percent level over the five-year period would be as follows:

Sequela	Difference Between No. at 95% and No. at 63%	Costs	Potential Savings
Stroke	90	$4,400	$396,000
Coronary heart disease	31	5,500	170,500
Cardiac failure	68	2,000	136,000
Renal impairment	37	5,000	185,000
			$887,500

This $887,500 represents a potential savings of $177,500 per year.

Discussion. Testing its original hypothesis of insufficient blood pressure control, the team found evidence of a potentially serious problem of patient management. Further study was necessary to verify these findings and to determine whether any of the factors involved was amenable to improvement. In view of the number of hypertensives out of control and of the serious prognostic implications for this patient group, no questions were raised about whether the standards applied were overly stringent, although the feasibility of eventually achieving blood pressure control in 95 percent of patients might be questioned.

Stage III: Definitive Assessment/Improvement Planning. This stage largely involves interpreting and supplementing data gathered in Stage II, to (1) validate the data from Stage II, (2) identify factors amenable to change that might correct the problem, and (3) establish a plan of action to solve it. Continuing our analogy to clinical management, we can say that Stage III consists in an analysis of the differential diagnosis so as to establish problem etiology and related factors for therapeutic planning. In conducting a quality assurance study, this means identifying not only the probable medical causes of deficient care but also the associated interpersonal relationships, organizational aspects, physician attitudes, and patient characteristics in terms of medical coping abilities and compliance. All these have contributed to the original problem and can influence the final improvement strategy.

Having found evidence of a potentially serious problem of patient management, the team undertook further study to verify these findings and to determine whether any of the factors involved was amenable to improvement. It was postulated that the noncontrol rate in excess of the standard could be explained by one of three alternatives: (1) inadequate therapeutic management by providers, (2) lack of compliance by patients in following the antihypertensive regimens, or (3) an invalid initial quality assessment study. Before any improvement action was advocated, the team decided to validate the initial findings and then to determine the cause of the excess in noncontrol.

1. *Methods.* To check the validity of the initial assessment findings, both study design and data were reanalyzed, and results of similar studies in other HMOs in the region were examined. Reanalysis of the original assessment data not only confirmed the high proportion of patients out of control but indicated that it was probably conservative in view of the criteria used. If 95 or 100 mm Hg diastolic pressure had been used as the indicator of control, over half the patients might have been considered "out of control." Comparisons of the study with related HMOs with similar patient populations revealed comparable findings, indicating that a patient management problem in fact very likely existed.

It had been decided that if the reanalysis confirmed the noncontrol rate, an objective written test developed to establish clinical knowledge of hypertension management (particularly chemotherapy) would be administered to the physicians to determine adequacy of therapeutic management. In addition, physicians would be tested to ascertain the accuracy of their judgment about the degree of compliance by their patients with the prescribed regimen. Since the reanalysis confirmed the existence of a problem, tests were administered to all fourteen primary care HMO physicians involved (mainly internists) to assess their clinical knowledge and their judgment on the issue of compliance.

It was also decided that a patient compliance test would be used to determine patients' knowledge of their condition, medication schedules, side effects of drugs, and probable effects of absence of treatment. Pill counts were also to be made to establish compliance in taking antihypertensive medication. Patients were then sent letters from their physicians informing them that they would be contacted by HMO quality assurance staff members to set up a series of appointments. It was explained that this program was not a research study but a systematic effort on the part of the HMO to improve benefits of the health care provided by the clinic. Over 50 percent of the patients responded favorably and set up a series of appointments with the quality assurance assistant; others, preferring to remain with their own physicians, retained their usual appointment schedule.

2. *Results.* Results of the physician questionnaire were as follows: (1) All the physicians accepted both the quality assessment design and the criteria used as valid and meaningful. (2) The test results showed that none of the physicians had inadequate pharmaceutical information regarding the management of patients with essential hypertension. (3) Ten of the fourteen physicians seriously overestimated the extent of their own patients' compliance with prescribed treatments. (4) Eleven of the physicians failed to mention patient health education as a component in their management of hypertensive patients.

Results from 148 patient questionnaires showed that (1) 15 percent were unaware that they were hypertensive or that their doctor was treating them for this problem; (2) 20 percent lacked information on the drug regimen prescribed by their doctor; (3) 81 percent could not state any side effects associated with the drugs they were taking; and (4) 93 percent did not know that there is little or no relation between symptoms and danger of uncontrolled high blood pressure. Moreover, 26 percent were not taking the medication prescribed, and 28 percent took their pills sporadically, mainly when they had headaches, which they attributed to their high blood pressure. In the aggregate, 95 percent were judged to have inadequate information about their condition, and 54 percent were obtaining inadequate medication.

Discussion. When initial assessment results do not meet standards, there are many possible explanations. It must always be kept in mind that it may be the assessment study that is deficient rather than the health care provided. Even where measurements are verified, however, other considerations may invalidate the findings. For example, it is possible that the standards are not realistic. Therefore, the definitive assessment stage must always include a reassessment of standards and a further confirmation of the assumption that improvement is possible.

Once deficiencies are verified, correctable determinants must be identified to permit improvement planning. An array of factors must be examined for improvement planning. Correctable determinants of care deficiencies may relate to providers, to patients, or to aspects of health care organization. In the case history described, the medical staff was convinced that care deficiencies uncovered in the initial assessment stage were real. The assessment findings confirmed studies (for example, Brook, 1974) relating to poor patient compliance. A controlled educational trial at Johns Hopkins (Inui, Yourtee, and Williamson, 1976) had demonstrated that physicians can indeed be taught to provide more adequate health outcomes (blood pressure control) in their patients. The quality assurance team concluded, therefore, that education factors had been identified that might be responsible for the high noncontrol rate measured and that these factors appeared amenable to improvement. In this case, both patients and physicians contributed to the problem. Accordingly, educational interventions to achieve improvement were required for both groups. The results of the patient and physician questionnaires provided the necessary details for designing a program of improvement for the identified deficiencies.

Stage IV: Implementing Improvement Actions. Stage IV requires implementing specific actions to accomplish the improvement that was judged feasible and was planned in Stage III. In our clinical patient management analogy, this function is equivalent to therapeutic action.

1. *Methods.* The quality assurance team was now ready to implement its agreed-on educational program with both providers and patients. A physician extender was hired as a quality assurance assistant at $20,000 a year and was authorized to establish a regular return visit schedule for hypertensive patients. The purpose of the return visits was to monitor blood pressure status, test patients' understanding of their disease, and provide education on possible complications and treatment, including the necessity to stay on medication and to be aware of possible toxic effects. Special emphasis was to be placed on ensuring that patients understood that

the dangers faced in hypertension have little relation to overt symptoms and that transitory symptoms such as headaches can be entirely unrelated to high blood pressure and certainly should not affect an antihypertensive regimen.

After surveying a range of health education materials that had been compiled, the staff felt that most of the materials were inappropriate for the specific needs of this group of patients. Therefore, some simple visual aids and questions to test patient understanding were designed, and special encounter forms were prepared to record the medication being taken. These materials were calculated to cost about $2,500 per year. A six-week revisit schedule was set up for patients who were out of control or indicated poor understanding of their problem.

On the basis of the questionnaire results and chart data, a second education program was designed for the physicians. This program provided information on the degree of therapeutic compliance by each physician's hypertensive patients. For those who requested it or showed inadequate understanding of the management of the essential hypertension patient, literature, such as that on controlled clinical trials conducted by the Veterans Administration Cooperative Study Group on Antihypertensive Agents (1967, 1970, 1972), was provided at a cost of $500 to the program.

2. *Results.* Patients who chose to visit the quality assurance assistant were very cooperative in responding to the questionnaires and to questions probing for understanding of their health problem. The visual aids proved successful once certain modifications were made; for example, it was necessary to translate them into Spanish to compensate for the language barrier. Patients' understanding improved, as was shown by the proportion who achieved better than 80 percent overall on the written questionnaire after several months of educational effort. Pill counts indicated apparent success in maintaining the prescribed medication schedules. Several patients who were not responding in terms of blood pressure control were referred to their physicians for a check and possible alteration of treatment. An unexpected result was an improvement in patient satisfaction and in provider/patient relationships. Many patients found it helpful to have someone listen to them about the stress of their daily life and often reported looking forward to the contacts with the quality assurance assistant.

Physician cooperation with the program was satisfactory, although at first there was some reluctance to take formal knowledge tests. A major accomplishment was that practically none of the physicians remained unaware of their patients' compliance problems. As a result, the physicians cooperated more fully with the quality assurance assistant by writing letters to their patients urging them to participate in the health education program and spending more time on patient health education during regular patient visits. Repeat testing after three months indicated that none of the physicians lacked understanding of or refused to accept health education as a therapeutic modality in the care of the hypertensive patient.

Discussion. Successful improvement programs require involvement of those responsible for improvement action in the planning process; valid problem formulation, which includes determining which factors and circumstances require special consideration; acceptable evidence that the specific improvement actions chosen will be effective; improvement measures that take into account local factors relating to the particular health care setting, patients, health problems, and involved providers; and frequent feedback during the improvement action process. However, even when these elements are present in the improvement program, it can still be difficult to provide adequate incentives for practitioners to alter their performance in response to a quality assessment study, as a recent review by Bertram and Brooks-Bertram (1977) shows.

The literature on adult learning shows that involvement of learners in identifying their own learning needs is important (Knox, 1977; Kidd, 1973). Therefore, quality assurance programs are more likely to be successful if as many staff members as possible are directly involved in formulating the assessment topics, designing the improvement plan, and evaluating the results. In this case, definitive assessment of hypertension control revealed an information gap that was correctable by educational measures involving both patients and physicians. Here, the educational program was adapted to the specific needs of each learner—probably a major reason for success—and the physicians were motivated to adopt the improvement action because they had been involved in the earlier stages (I, II, and III) of the study as well.

During the improvement stage of a quality assurance study, specific feedback is useful to determine whether the improvement plan needs to be modified. In the case in question, the results of the brief tests of knowledge administered to both physicians and patients resulted in an educational diagnosis on which learning prescriptions could be written. However, this continual improvement in performance, though helpful for planning the educational program, was not yet indicative of the ultimate success or failure of the project. To determine the impact of the quality assurance program, measurements of health outcomes in the patients (blood pressure control) were required.

Stage V: Reassessment. Stage V, the final step in this process, involves reassessing the results of the preceding stages with a view to determining whether and to what extent desired goals have been accomplished. This is analogous to the return visit and/or recheck of laboratory results of the therapy in clinical practice. It allows the team to evaluate the results of improvement actions and establish evidence that significant changes are in fact related to the quality assurance actions taken. This step is frequently neglected and may be difficult to undertake. It is important because it alone can provide a factual basis for planning further action.

Six months after the educational program had been in progress, the quality assurance team undertook its reassessment to determine whether any improvement in hypertension control had occurred.

1. *Methods.* A sampling of the original group of patients was conducted.

2. *Results.* A marked change in health problem status was found: The overall rate of noncontrol had dropped from 36 to 19 percent, a statistically significant improvement, although still four times the standard of 5 percent set at the outset of the quality assurance study. The group of 148 patients who made regular appointments with the quality assurance assistant achieved twice the improvement observed for the 100 patients who had insisted on seeing only their own physicians for help in controlling their hypertension. In percentage terms, improvement in the latter group was almost identical to that measured by Inui, Yourtee, and Williamson (1976) in a controlled educational trial in which patient health edu-

cation about hypertension was offered only by the physicians providing care.

Given the acceptable evidence of improved blood pressure control, it was then necessary to determine whether the change in this group of patients could be attributed to the improvement actions. An outside group supervising the study rechecked the data and data-collection method and indicated that the improved blood pressure findings were valid. The increase in the control rate of the patients seeing only their physicians seemed reasonable in view of the data from the controlled trial. In other words, there was evidence that teaching physicians better skills in patient health education can have a beneficial effect on specific, measured health outcomes. The even greater improvement for patients also seen by a quality assurance assistant and instructed in aspects of compliance with prescribed regimens may reflect the effectiveness of this specific improvement modality, an assumption supported by controlled studies of patient compliance by Sackett and Haynes (1976). It could not be determined, however, whether the significantly greater improvement in the group monitored by the quality assurance assistant was entirely due to the improvement program, which involved more frequent visits and possibly stress management as well. It may have been due in part to self-selection of a more compliant or less severely ill group of patients and to the specific health problems involved.

At this point in the process, the team had shown, by repeat study, that efforts had been successful in raising the level of hypertensive patients under control to 81 percent, still short of the 95 percent goal. Re-cycling to Stage III, the team accepted the hypothesis that continued efforts to strengthen physician education and patient education would lead to more improvement in results. This improvement was accomplished during the ensuing year (Stage IV) and required an additional expenditure of $2,000 for AV materials.

In August 1976, an assessment study was once again repeated (Stage V). The results from this analysis revealed a 91 percent level of control—still not at the 95 percent goal, but rapidly approaching it. At this point, the team conducted another careful survey to ascertain whether extraneous factors other than increased efforts at education might have contributed to the latest improvement. No other plausible factors were discovered, and therefore attribution was placed on the education effort.

Discussion. Several conclusions can be drawn at the final stage in a quality assurance cycle. It is at this point that the results of reassessment should be examined to determine whether additional expenditure of resources is justified, taking into account potential for further improvement in a particular problem area.

• *Conclusion 1.* Evidence acceptable to providers and observers of the impact of quality assurance must be obtained. In the best case, reassessment of the original problem should be completed in the final stage of a quality assurance study to determine whether significant improvement has been achieved and standards have been met. As a minimum, consensus among qualified observers should be obtained to determine whether benefits achieved seem worth the effort expended.

In this case history, data were obtained to determine impact. It should be noted, however, that this case presents an example of a degree of effort and perseverance by the assessment team that cannot be taken for granted in all settings.

• *Conclusion 2.* If improvement is confirmed, acceptable evidence should be established that the observed changes are due to the quality assurance measures that were taken. In the best case, documentation of efficacy of improvement modalities established in controlled trials reported in the literature should be obtained. As a minimum, consensus of a group of qualified observers should be obtained regarding possible alternative explanations for any improvement observed.

In this case, reasonable evidence of attribution was secured. The team knew of a documented controlled study (Inui, Yourtee, and Williamson, 1976) that had determined the efficacy of education in improving patient compliance and health outcomes. On the basis of that study and data from their assessment studies, the team members could be reasonably sure that the improvement noted was due to the action they had taken.

In this instance, evidence was obtained suggesting an association between the measured improvement and the actions taken. This type of evidence is rarely established for any education program (Bertram and Brooks-Bertram, 1977), let alone for the clinical management of patients. On the one hand, physicians often do not know what eventually happens to their patients in terms of health problem control when the patient does not return. On the other hand, when subsequent examination reveals improvement, it is usual to assume that therapeutic management was responsible for the changes noted. This may or may not be a valid assumption, and one of the major functions of quality assurance programs is to stimulate providers to question such assumptions.

• *Conclusion 3.* The cost of the quality assurance effort must be estimated and weighed against the value of the impact achieved. In the best case, careful unit costing of all related direct and indirect costs by qualified accountants and analysis by an economist should be obtained. As a minimum, consensual cost estimates by a group of qualified observers should be weighed against the extent of confirmed improvement.

An economic analysis of the case study can be summarized as follows. Considering the HMO enrollee population of 2,520 with mild to severe hypertension, the team had estimated that, at the 63 percent control rate revealed in the first study, the HMO could expect, over the next five years, the following hospitalizations secondary to hypertension:

Sequela	No.	Cost/Hospitalization	Total
Stroke	170	$4,400	$ 748,000
Coronary heart disease	186	5,500	1,023,000
Cardiac failure	78	2,000	156,000
Renal impairment	56	5,000	280,000
		Current costs:	$2,207,000

At a 95 percent control rate, which was the quality assurance goal, the HMO could expect, over the next five years, the following hospitalizations secondary to hypertension:

Sequela	No.	Cost/Hospitalization	Total
Stroke	80	4,400	$ 352,000
Coronary heart disease	155	5,500	852,500
Cardiac failure	10	2,000	20,000
Renal impairment	19	5,000	95,000
		Achievable costs:	$1,319,500

The difference between the costs of hospitalizations at the 95 percent and 63 percent control levels represents a savings to the HMO of $887,500 over five years, or $177, 500 a year.

However, some of these savings would be offset by the costs of the improvement actions taken as part of the quality assurance effort. For example, the HMO was now investing the following amounts in quality assurance and cost containment efforts:

Estimated yearly cost of quality assurance and cost containment team efforts	$ 1,500
Salary and fringe benefits for quality assurance assistant	20,000
Physician education	500
AV materials (first year)	1,500
Additional AV materials (second year)	2,000
Total	$25,500

Nevertheless, if the education program resulted in the projected 95 percent success rate, the HMO would still realize a significant potential savings.

$177,500 estimated savings/year (at the 95 percent success rate)
− 25,500 expenditures/year on quality assurance effort
$152,000 net savings/year

If only the 91 percent success rate achieved at the end of the second year could be maintained over the five-year period, the hospitalizations secondary to hypertension were predicted to be as follows:

Sequela	No.	Cost/Hospitalization	Total
Stroke	98	$4,400	$ 431,200
Coronary heart disease	164	5,500	902,000
Cardiac failure	19	2,000	38,000
Renal impairment	25	5,000	125,000
			$1,496,200

Comparing these costs with those that would be incurred at the 63 percent control level ($2,207,000), it is evident that over the five-year period there would still be a significant savings to the HMO of $710,800 ($142,160/year), although some $45,000 a year less than at the 95 percent level. This savings would be offset by the cost of the quality assurance program as follows:

$142,160 estimated savings/year (at 91 percent success rate)
— 25,500 expenditures/year for quality assurance effort
$116,660 net savings/year

This analysis considered only the direct cost-savings benefits to the HMO. Other factors need to be considered in assessing the benefits of the quality assurance effort. First, should the cost per hospitalization increase more rapidly than the yearly cost of the program, obviously the potential savings would increase correspondingly each year. However, since the dollar amounts attached to this economic analysis represent only potential savings, and since the HMO will, of course, attempt to have all its hypertensive enrollees under control (that is, there will be no definitive study with nontreated "controls"), the HMO will not be able to measure precisely the cost benefit. Moreover, these savings would accrue to the HMO and its enrollees collectively (that is, potentially, all enrollees would benefit whether or not they were hypertensive) and only to this HMO. Any savings associated with reduced hospital use for an isolated health problem may not necessarily accrue to society at large if the reduced hospitalization rate does not result in a concurrent overall reduction in hospital resource utilization. In other words, the reduced hospital rate for this HMO might be picked up by another group with increasing utilization; or society in general may end up paying higher hospitalization rates per admission if the hospitals' fixed expenditures are not otherwise reduced.

A hypertension control program such as the one described in this case can produce benefits and costs other than those just discussed. For example, benefits to patients and families could include

- Savings of direct treatment costs of extended care facilities, home nursing, medications, and rehabilitation services.
- Savings of potential earnings losses and opportunity losses resulting from disability or death.
- Avoidance of potential health loss, such as pain, suffering, disability, and anxiety.

Other benefits to the HMO could include

- Improved goodwill and improved marketing capability of the HMO, particularly if the results of the quality assurance efforts are documented and distributed.
- Improved satisfaction among HMO personnel as they realize concrete results from their quality assurance and cost containment efforts.

However, such a program imposes additional potential costs on both patients and physicians. For example, it is possible that the intensive patient education efforts to attain 95 percent control of hypertension through compliance with the regimen prescribed by the HMO clinician will cause some patient dissatisfaction with loss of "individual freedom." In like manner, the necessity for all clinicians to pursue this goal may engender some concern or dissatisfaction among the clinicians about loss of "autonomy."

It may be difficult to place precise dollar values on each of these additional benefits and costs. However, with careful analysis and application of a relative value scale, each can be included in the final program evaluation. Stason and Weinstein have provided an excellent review of cost-effective analysis for health and medical practices and noteworthy commentary on the allocation of resources to manage hypertension (Stason and Weinstein, 1977).

Summary

The five stages of a quality assurance study, which encompasses cost containment, have been presented through the use of an illustrative case history based in part on an actual quality assurance project. This case showed the relations between a quality assurance program used to ensure improved preventive services and the eventual health care cost savings. It also demonstrated the five generic stages of a quality assurance study based on a problem-solving approach. This problem-oriented strategy is now required of hospitals throughout the United States to meet the quality assurance requirements and regulations of both the Joint Commission on Accreditation of Hospitals (JCAH) and the Professional Standards Review Organizations (PSROs). By understanding the basic similarity of such a strategy to clinical problem solving, future health care professionals will have a strong theoretical framework for assessing and improving their future practice. This approach may well provide essential adaptive resources for more successful coping with this modern era of accelerating technological and social change.

Self-Evaluation Exercises

1. Identify the stages of quality assurance that were completed in this study and discuss the approach used in each stage.
2. Review the five types of information required for selecting topics for quality assurance study (importance, efficacy, effectiveness, efficiency, improvement potential). Give evidence from the case that the information obtained indicated that this health problem warranted assessment and improvement.
3. Consider the standard set by the quality assurance team. What evidence is there that this standard was appropriate? Inappropriate?
4. Identify unforeseen factors that may have contributed to the improvement in outcome among both physicians and patients. Discuss implications of these factors for future practice.
5. The team considered four other topics for study—management of urinary tract infections in females, follow-up of abnormal laboratory findings in general, use of skull roentgenogram in minor head injury, and management of otitis media in children. Select one. Describe an acceptable standard of maximum acceptable deficiency and then document the validity of the standard by consulting the literature.

       Identify factors to be measured to compare actual performance with standards.

6.   Using the topic selected in Question 5, discuss the achievable health benefits to be gained and the potential cost savings from a successful quality assurance effort.

7.   Design an improvement plan. (Reminder: Information acquired in completing Question 5 must be taken into consideration.)

8.   Prognosticate the results of the improvement actions in terms of health benefits and cost savings and design a plan for reassessing the results of the quality assurance effort.

9.   Return to the case study presented as an exercise for self-evaluation at the end of Chapter Three. Critique this case on the basis of the information from the five-stage case study presented in this chapter.

Appendix A

Sources of National and Local Data on Health Problems

ᴥᴥᴥᴥᴥᴥᴥᴥᴥᴥᴥᴥᴥᴥᴥᴥᴥᴥᴥᴥᴥᴥᴥ

I. **Frequency of Health Problems and Magnitude of Disabilities (Health Loss) in the United States**

    A. *National Data* (Available from Federal Agencies)

        Several publications on these topics are available from:

            Office of Health Research, Statistics, and Technology
            National Center for Health Statistics
            Public Health Service

Dept. of Health and Human Services
Hyattsville MD 20782[1]

These include the following periodic reports:

1. *Vital and Health Statistics* in the following series:

   Series 10—*Data from the Health Interview Surveys*

   These reports, based on data collected in a continuing national household interview survey, give statistics on illness, accidental injuries, disability, and use of hospital, medical, dental, and other services.

   Examples

   #111—*Limitations of Activity Due to Chronic Conditions. Results of National Household Survey, 1974.*[2]

   This report summarizes the characteristics of patients and extent of disability related to thirty common chronic health problems.

   #125—*Acute Conditions, Incidence and Associated Disability, U.S., July 1976–June 1977.* Publication No. (PHS) 78-1554.

   Provides tables on incidence of acute conditions and degree of bed disability, associated days of restricted activity, and time lost from work and school in U.S. population according to sex, age, color, calendar quarter, place of incident, and geographic region.

[1]To obtain a copy of the Current Listing and Topical Index to the Vital and Health Statistics Series and the Catalogue of Publications of NCHS, write to: Scientific and Technical Information Branch, National Center for Health Statistics, Public Health Service, 3700 East-West Highway, Hyattsville MD 20782.
[2]Data from these tables were used to augment the case study developed for this text.

Series 11—*Data from the Health Examination Survey*

These periodic reports provide data from direct examination, testing, and measurement of national samples of the civilian, noninstitutionalized U.S. population.

Examples

#166—*Cardiovascular Conditions of Children 6–11 Years and Youths 12–17 Years, U.S., 1963–1965 and 1966–1970.* Publication No. (PHS) 78-1653.

#203—*Blood Pressure Levels of Persons 6–74 Years, U.S., 1971–1974.* J. Roberts and K. Maurer. Publication No. (HRA) 78-1648.[3]

Series 13—*Data on Health Resource Utilization*

These periodic reports provide statistics on the utilization of health manpower and facilities providing long-term care, ambulatory care, hospital care, and family planning services. They are derived from the following ongoing surveys:

- National Ambulatory Medical Care Survey
- National Hospital Discharge Survey
- National Nursing Home Survey
- National Reporting System for Family Planning Services

Example

#44—*National Ambulatory Medical Care Survey, 1977 Summary.* Publication No. (PHS) 80-1795.[4]

[3]These data were included to augment the case history used in this text.

[4]For an example of the type of analyses of practice styles using these data, see Noren, J., and others, "Ambulatory Medical Care. A Comparison of Internists and Family-General Physicians," *New England Journal of Medicine*, 1980, *302*(1), 11–16.

Provides data on types and frequency of health problems on a national basis, using statistical data obtained from a national sample of office-based physicians on the provision and utilization of ambulatory medical care in physicians' offices during 1977. Hospital ambulatory clinics, public health clinics, and federal ambulatory care visits are not included in this sample.

Series 20—*Data on Mortality*

These reports contain data on mortality in the United States, with special analyses by cause of death, age, and other demographic variables and geographic and time series analyses.

2. *Publications on Health Indexes*

These provide frequent reports on newly developing methodologies to measure health indexes (a measure of disability) on a yearly and quarterly basis.

Example

Clearinghouse on Health Indexes—Cumulated Annotations, 1976. Publication No. (PHS) 78-1225.

Contains an annotation of articles on health indexes in 1976 and is useful as a resource on various methodologies, although it contains no national aggregate data. Portions of this document were printed during the year on a quarterly basis and labeled as supplement to (PHS) 78-1225.

3. *Periodic Reviews of General Statistical Information on Health*

Example

Facts at Your Fingertips—A Guide to Sources of Statistical Information on Major Health Topics. (3rd

ed.) Fall 1978. National Center for Health
Statistics, Hyattsville, Md. Publication No.
(PHS) 79-1246. Available at National Technical
Information Service, U.S. Department of
Commerce, Springfield VA 22161, HRP
0029568.

Cites a listing of papers on health topics from
"Accidents" to "Visual disorders." It is not intended to be complete or comprehensive but
does provide some very useful leads to finding national data on incidence of and disability due to various health problems.

B. *National Data* (Available in the Private Sector)

1. *The Rand Health Insurance Study*

This study contains reports of a social experiment
supported by a grant from the U.S. Department of
Health and Human Services to investigate the effects
of different health care financing arrangements on
use of health services, quality of care, satisfaction,
and health status. In that portion of the study related
to health status, Rand researchers have (1) developed
methods to measure health status and (2) reported
some preliminary results in the measurement on
some of the six experimental sites. The following is a
listing of individual reports that contain useful information on health status of selected populations
within the United States.

Examples

Ware, J. E., Jr., Brook, R. H., Williams, K. N.,
Stewart, A. L., and Davies-Avery, A. Vol. I,
Model of Health and Methodology, R-1987/1-HEW.

Stewart, A. L., Ware, J. E., Jr., Brook, R. H., and
Davies-Avery, A. Vol. II, *Physical Health in Terms
of Functioning,* R-1987/2-HEW.

Ware, J. E., Jr., Johnston, S. A., Davies-Avery, A., and Brook, R. H. Vol. III, *Mental Health*, R-1987/3-HEW.

Donald, C. A., Ware, J. E., Jr., Brook, R. H., and Davies-Avery, A. Vol. IV, *Social Health*, R-1987/4-HEW.

Ware, J. E., Jr., Davies-Avery, A., and Donald, C. A. Vol. V, *General Health Perceptions*, R-1987/5-HEW.

Ware, J. E., Jr., Brook, R. H., and Davies-Avery, A. Vol. VI, *Analysis of Relationships Among Health Status Measures*, R-1987/6-HEW.

Rogers, W. H., Williams, K. N., and Brook, R. H. Vol. VII, *Power Analysis of Health Status Measures*, R-1987/7-HEW.

Brook, R. H., Ware, J. E., Jr., Davies-Avery, A., Stewart, A. L., Donald, C. A., Rogers, W. H., Williams, K. N., and Johnston, S. A. Vol. VIII, *Overview*, R-1987/8-HEW.[5]

Eisen, M., Donald, C. A., Ware, J. E., Jr., and Brook, R. H. Conceptualization and Measurement of *Health for Children* in the Health Insurance Study, The Rand Corporation, R-2313-HEW.

2.   *Reports of the American Medical Association*

The American Medical Association provides yearly tabulation of physician practice profiles.

Examples

Profile of Medical Practice 1978 (revised yearly). American Medical Association, Center for

[5] Also appears as Brook, R. H., and others. "Overview of Adult Health Status Measures Fielded in Rand's Health Insurance Study," *Medical Care*, 1979, *17*(7) (Supplement).

Health Services Research and Development, Order Department OP-52, P.O. Box 821, Monroe WI 53566.

Contains tabulations of data on physician manpower by geographic and specialty distribution, physician/population ratios, physician work patterns (hours of work per week, patients seen per day, and so on), physician fees and income, as well as selected papers on health care cost management. Does not provide specific data on types of health problems.

C. *Local Data*

A number of yearly publications on this topic are available from:

Office of Statistical Research
National Center for Health Statistics
Public Health Service
Dept. of Health and Human Services
Hyattsville MD 20782

1. *Federal compilations of local data*

   Examples

   State Estimates of Disability and Utilization of Medical Services: U.S. 1974–1976. Publication No. (PHS) 78-1241.

   Contains data on disability from acute and chronic conditions, home confinement, short-stay hospitalizations, and physician and dentist visits on a state-by-state basis.

   Model State Vital Statistics Act and Model State Vital Statistics Regulations. May 1978. Publication No. (PHS) 78-1115.

Contains no data but is designed for use by state registrars of vital statistics and state legislators to promote uniformity of policies and procedures to enhance the level of comparability of vital statistics among the various states and to minimize duplication.

2. *State-generated data*

   Example

   The 1973 Michigan Ambulatory Medical Care Survey, May 1973–April 1974. March 1976. Cornell, R., Ozgoren, F., and Rutherford, J. Department of Biostatistics, School of Public Health, University of Michigan.

   Presents statistics on the use of office-based physician services by ambulatory patients based on data from the Michigan Ambulatory Medical Care Survey of 1973. This survey is an augmentation of the National Ambulatory Medical Care Survey that enables Michigan data to be presented separately. The results of these data indicate that Michigan State data do not differ significantly from national ambulatory data. This may be of interest to those questioning the extrapolation of national data to local conditions. Preliminary data for the city of Detroit indicate rather marked differences from national or state totals, however.

II. **Costs and Resource Expenditures for Health Conditions (Direct and Indirect Economic Costs)**

A. *National Data*

   A large number of publications are available from:

   Office of Health Research, Statistics, and Technology
   National Center for Health Statistics

Public Health Service
Dept. of Health and Human Services
Hyattsville MD 20782

These include the following periodic reports:

1. *Vital and Health Statistics* in the following series:

    Series 10—*Data from the Health Interview Surveys*

    Example

    #122—Personal Out-of-Pocket Health Expenses, U.S., 1975. Publication No. (PHS) 79-1550.

    Series 13—*Data on Health Resources Utilization*

    Examples

    #38—Nursing Home Costs, U.S. National Nursing Home Survey, August 1973–April 1974. Publication No. (PHS) 79-1789.

    #41—Utilization of Short-Stay Hospitals, Annual Summary of the United States, 1977. B. J. Haupt. Publication No. (PHS) 79-1792.

    Detailed Diagnoses and Surgical Procedures for Patients Discharged from Short-Stay Hospitals: United States, 1977.[6] Publication No. (PHS) 79-1274.

    Displays hospitalization use in terms of numbers and rates of first-listed diagnosis, of days of care, and of operations performed. Published to improve access to the medical data available from the National

---

[6]For a review of the evolution of hospital-discharge data systems in the United States and what is known about the quality of such data, see *Reliability of National Discharge Survey Data,* 1980, ISBN 0-309-03079-X 1980. Institute of Medicine, National Academy of Sciences, National Academy Press, 2101 Constitution Avenue NW, Washington, DC 20418. It analyzes a defined sample of the medical records of the NHDS file for 1977 and compares the reliability of this information with data from private abstracting services and the Health Care Financing Administration.

Hospital Discharge Survey (NHDS) of the National Center for Health Statistics (NCHS). Data for newborns are excluded from this report.

2. *Annual Comprehensive Reports of the National Center for Health Services Research and National Center for Health Statistics*

These federal agencies jointly produce reports on recent trends in the health sector and detailed discussions of selected current health issues.

Examples

Health. United States, 1979. National Center for Health Statistics, National Center for Health Services Research, Public Health Service, Dept. of Health, Education, and Welfare, Hyattsville MD 20782. Publication No. (PHS) 80-1232.

Contains statistics on health status and determinants (birth rates, death rates, life expectancy rates, disability by disease or health problem); utilization of health resources by manpower and facilities; and health expenditures. The comprehensive, detailed data herein fulfill a statutory requirement that the Secretary of HHS compile periodic reports on the health of the population, utilization of health resources, health care costs, and financing, acting through the NCHSR and the NCHS with advice of the U.S. National Committee on Vital and Health Statistics.

3. *National Medical Care Expenditure Survey*[7]

[7] To be placed on their mailing list, write:
National Medical Care Expenditure Survey
Public Health Service OASH
Room 1-57, Center Bldg.
3700 East-West Highway
Hyattsville MD 20782

Data Previews

Example

#1—Announcement of National Medical Care Expenditures Survey Publications, October 11, 1978.

Contains data from: (1) household survey; (2) physician and hospital survey; and (3) employees and insurance companies survey. These survey populations are sampled so as to be representative of the entire nation. "Will represent one of the most comprehensive bodies of information ever assembled for a one-year period on the health care experiences of the American people."

4. *Reports of the Health Care Financing Administration*

This agency distributes provider data on use of health services by Medicaid and Medicare recipients.

Example

The *Social Security Bulletin,* published monthly, provides data on types of expenditures and source of funds. Such data dramatically illustrate the economic importance of the health industry to both the national economy and the population at large. For example, a complete review of health care expenditures for fiscal year 1977 appeared in the July 1978 issue.

Deacon, R. "Impact of Medicare on the Use of Medical Services by Disabled Beneficiaries 1972–74." *Health Care Financing Review,* Fall 1979, pp. 39–54.

Presents an analysis of data collected through the current Medicare survey on medical services used both before and after coverage. Contains data on types of disabilities and costs for services.

Hsiao, W., and Stason, W. "Toward Developing a Relative Value Scale for Medical and Surgical Services." *Health Care Financing Review,* Fall 1979, pp. 23–38.

> Presents a method to determine the relative values of surgical procedures and medical office visits on the basis of resource costs.

Health Care Financing Trends. Fall 1979, Vol. 1, No. 1. Published quarterly by HCFA's Office of Research, Demonstrations and Statistics.

> Provides tables of national data on total health expenditures, selected community hospital statistics from the National Hospital Panel Survey, medical care prices including annual percentage change in average medical care consumer price indexes, employment and earnings in health care sector, national economic indicators, and listings of contacts for further information.

Health Care Financing Notes.

> Provides the public with descriptive information as soon as it becomes available. These reports are published irregularly; frequently a more comprehensive analysis of the data may be available later in one of HCFA's other publications.

Medicare: Use of Home Health Services, 1978.

> Contains tables of data on number of home visits and accounts of charges to Medicare recipients by region and contains patient demographics.

Health Care Financing Program Statistics (published monthly).[8] Preliminary National Monthly Medicaid Statistics.

Presents data on total amount of medical payments under Title XIX by form of payment and reporting states, and basis of eligibility of recipients.

5. *Studies by Rice, Cooper, Mushkin, Berk, Paringer, and Associates*

Examples

Rice, D. *Estimating the Cost of Illness.* Health Economics Series No. 6. U.S. Public Health Service, 1966.

Contains numerous tabulations of data on health care costs and represents the first major effort to estimate the costs of illness in the United States in 1963.

Cooper, B., and Rice, D. "The Economic Cost of Illness Revisited." *Social Security Bulletin,* February 1976.

Updates the original 1963 data estimates, using more current cost information and improved data, which enabled a more sophisticated approach.

Mushkin, S., Paringer, L., and Berk, A. *Costs of Illness and Disease, Fiscal Year 1975.* Public Services Laboratory (PSL) of Georgetown University under Contract #N01-OD-5-2121. Division of Program Analysis, NIH.[9]

[8]To obtain copies of this and other publications of HCFA, write to:
ORDS Publications
Room 1E9, Oak Meadows Bldg.
6340 Security Blvd.
Baltimore MD 21235
[9]National Technical Information Service
U.S. Dept. of Commerce
Springfield VA 22161
NIH 74-7/9-1, PB 280 298

Contains detailed tabulations on health care expenditures, economic losses, and productivity losses related to illness for 1975.

Berk, A., and Paringer, L. *Costs of Illness and Disease, Fiscal Year 1930.* Public Services Laboratory (PSL) of Georgetown University. Under Contract No. NO1-OD-S-2121. Division of Program Analysis, NIH.[10]

Examines the costs of illness in the United States in 1930, using the same methodology as the 1975 report. From this one can make comparisons over a forty-five-year time span.

Mushkin, S., Paringer, L., and Berk, A. *Costs of Illness and Disease, 1900.* Public Services Laboratory (PSL) of Georgetown University. Under Contract No. 1-OD-5-2121. Division of Program Analysis, NIH.[11]

Presents estimates of direct health expenditures of morbidity costs and/or mortality costs by disease category for the year 1900, using methodology for estimating costs for 1975.

Mushkin, S., and others. *Costs of Disease and Illness in the U.S. in the Year 2000.* Public Services Laboratory (PSL) of Georgetown University. Under Contract No. NO1-OD-S-2121. Division of Program Analysis, NIH.[12]

[10]National Technical Information Service
U.S. Dept. of Commerce
Springfield VA 22161
NIH 74-1/9-2 PB 280-299
[11]National Technical Information Service
U.S. Dept. of Commerce
Springfield VA 22161
NIH 74-7/9-3 PB 280-300
[12]*Public Health Reports,* Special Supplement, 1978, *93*(5), 495-588.

Projects the cost of illness to the year 2000, a reasonable benchmark for long-range planning, and presents numerous tables on projected direct and indirect costs.

B. *Incidental Reports*

Examples

Acton, J. *Measuring the Social Impact of Heart and Circulatory Disease Programs: Preliminary Framework and Estimates.* The Rand Corporation. Santa Monica, Calif. 90406. April 1975. R-1697-NHLI.[13]

Contains detailed national data on morbidity, mortality, and medical costs of various heart and circulatory diseases, including acute-hospital costs, earnings lost, and human capital loss. It presents a quantification of the principal elements of social effects of illness and gives two alternative measures of their net value, one based on the livelihood-saving (or human capital) approach and the other on individualistic preferences (or willingness to pay).

Acton, J. *Evaluating Public Programs to Save Lives: The Case of Heart Attacks.* The Rand Corporation. Santa Monica, Calif. 90406. January 1973. R-950-RC.

Presents a method for evaluating health programs by structuring the problem as a decision-making exercise and applying a willingness-to-pay measure of the worth of the program.

Luft, H., Bunker, J., and Enthoven, A. "Should Operations Be Regionalized? The Empirical Rela-

[13]Data from this paper were used in the hypothetical case study developed for this text.

tion Between Surgical Volume and Mortality." *New England Journal of Medicine*, 1979, *301*(25), 1364–1369.

Examines and presents data on the mortality rates for twelve surgical procedures of varying complexity in 1,498 hospitals to determine whether there is a relation between a hospital's surgical volume and its surgical mortality.

Kridel, R., and Winston, D. *Cost Effective Medical Care. A Guide on Cost Consciousness for Physicians in Training.* Work Group of Cost Effective Medical Care. Resident Physicians Section, American Medical Association, Chicago, 1978.

Presents some national data on health care expenditures and describes some cost containment programs in individual hospitals that centered on defining costs of individual services, procedures, and so on.

Rice, D., Feldman, J., and White, K. "The Current Burden of Illness in the U.S." Occasional paper. Institute of Medicine, National Academy of Sciences, Washington, D.C. Presented at annual meeting of Institute of Medicine, October 27, 1976. 36 pp.

Provides tables of national data by disease category on potential years of life lost, distribution of inpatient days, physician office visits, work-loss days, major activity limitations, and distribution of direct and indirect economic costs by illness.

Fielding, J. "Role of Data in the Assessment of Quality of Hospital Care in the Professional Standards Review Organizations." In *Proceedings of the 15th National Meeting of Public Health Conference on Records and Statistics.* DHEW Publication No. (HRA) 75-1214.

Advancing the Quality of Health Care. A Policy Statement. Institute of Medicine, National Academy of Sciences. August 1974. IOM Publication 74-04.

Recommends that data used for quality assurance purposes be problem-oriented, specific to recipients of care and providers, population-based, period-explicit, and place-specific. This report suggests methods for collecting and retrieving uniform data and methods to ensure compatability of all health care data, describing the role of NCHS in this process.

Appendix B

Federal Sources of National Data on Efficacy

ʝʚʝʚʝʚʝʚʝʚʝʚʝʚʝʚʝʚʝʚʝʚʝʚʝʚʝʚʝʚʝʚʝʚʝʚ

I. **Reports of the National Center for Health Care Technology (NCHCT)[1]**

This center was created to set priorities for technology assessment (efficacy studies) and to encourage, conduct, and support assessments, research, demonstrations, and evalua-

[1]See Perry, S., and Kalberer, J. "The NIH Consensus Development Program and the Assessment of Health Care Technologies: The First Two Years." *New England Journal of Medicine,* 1980, *103* (3), 169–172.

tions concerning health care technology. However, it has been defunded. For information on results of studies so far completed, write:

National Center for Health Care Technology
5600 Fishers Lane, Parklawn Building
Rockville MD 20857

II. Reports of the National Institutes of Health

A. Office of Medical Applications of Research (OMAR)[2]

This agency, located in the Office of the Director, National Institutes of Health (NIH), is the focal point of a program aimed at improving the translation of the results of biomedical research pertinent to health care into knowledge that can be effectively employed in the practice of medicine and public health. In carrying out this function, OMAR facilitates and coordinates technical consensus development activities at the NIH. These activities involve biomedical researchers, practicing professionals, and others in the exchange of information and opinions on the suitability for general application of emerging health care technologies or those already in general use. Much of the discussion relates to known efficacy studies or the future design of appropriate efficacy studies. For information about the Consensus Development Program and for summaries of conferences held to date, write:

Charles U. Lowe, M.D.
Acting NIH Associate Director for Medical
    Applications of Research
Office of Medical Applications of Research
National Institutes of Health
Bldg. 1, Room 216
Bethesda MD 20205

[2]See Perry, S. "The Biomedical Research Community: Its Place in Consensus Development." *Journal of the American Medical Association,* 1978, *239* (5), 5–9.

III. Reports of the Office of Technology — U.S. Congress

The congressional Office of Technology Assessment was asked by the Senate Committee on Human Resources "to examine federal policies and current medical practices to determine whether a reasonable amount of justification should be provided before costly new medical technologies and procedures are put into general use." Consequently, a series of authoritative studies is being conducted, and the following reports have been published:

A. *Development of Medical Technology: Opportunities for Assessment.* August 1976.

Focuses on assessment of the societal impact of medical technologies.

B. *Policy Implications of the Computed Tomography (CT) Scanner.* August 1978.

Examines the effects of public and private policies on the development, diffusion, use, and reimbursement of CT scanners.

C. *Assessing the Efficacy and Safety of Medical Technologies.* September 1978.

Examines the importance and current status of information on efficacy and safety as well as techniques and programs for generating this information. (Much of the efficacy reference material in this text was abstracted from this excellent source.)

D. *The Implications of Cost-Effectiveness Analysis of Medical Technology.* August 1980.

Analyzes the feasibility, implications, and usefulness of cost-effectiveness and cost benefit analysis in health care decision making.

Copies of the above reports can be obtained from:

Congress of the United States
Office of Technology Assessment
Washington DC 20510

or

Superintendent of Documents
U.S. Government Printing Office
Washington DC 20402

IV. Reports of the Food and Drug Administration

The Food and Drug Administration (FDA) of the Department of Health and Human Services (HHS, formerly HEW) has responsibility for protecting the health of the American public in the areas of foods, drugs, veterinary medicine, x-ray equipment, radiation-emitting medical and consumer devices, blood banks, vaccines and allergenics, organ transplants, and other biological products.

A. Prescription Drugs

The FDA is required to approve the efficacy and safety of all new drugs before they are marketed. Although regulation of drug safety has been required since the Food, Drug and Cosmetic Act of 1938, the requirement regarding efficacy has been in effect only since 1962.

The Drug Efficacy Study Implementation (DESI) project was organized to evaluate the efficacy of the approximately 3,500 drugs marketed between 1938 and 1962 and approved only for safety. Expert teams were organized for each drug family to evaluate efficacy, using consensual group methods.

The results of this FDA study (assisted by the National Academy of Science/National Research Council) categorizes efficacy in four classes: (1) ineffective, (2) possibly effective, (3) probably effective, and (4) effective.

The efficacy results are reported in the "FDA Trade Name Index of All Prescription Drugs in the DESI Project," obtainable from:

U.S. Food and Drug Administration
5600 Fishers Lane
Rockville MD 20857
Attention: HFD-32

B.   Medical Devices

In the Food, Drug and Cosmetic Act of 1938, the FDA had to prove that a product was in fact dangerous or fraudulent before any action would be taken to remove it from the market. The Medical Devices Act of 1976 extends the authority of the FDA to evaluation of efficacy and safety to be made "weighing any probable benefit to health from use of the device against any risk of injury or illness from such use." Examples of devices include optical prescription lenses/frames, hearing aids, intrauterine devices, surgical instruments, cardiac pacemakers, CT scanners, and "in vitro diagnostic products." There are likely over 8,000 such devices encompassed by this act. Nineteen panels of experts have been created to recommend efficacy groupings in three classes:

Class I   Devices need only meet "Good Manufacturing Practices" (GMP) regulations.

Class II   Devices must meet specific performance standards developed by the FDA or specified outside institutions. Criteria for sensitivity, accuracy, materials, safety, and durability are included.

Class III   Devices must undergo a process of premarket approval based on substantial research evidence of efficacy and safety.

V. Other Federal Sources of Efficacy Data and Information

A. Alcohol, Drug Abuse, and Mental Health Administration (ADAMHA)

Three components have conducted research on efficacy and safety of medical technologies since the 1950s: the National Institute on Alcohol Abuse and Alcoholism (NIAAA), the National Institute on Drug Abuse (NIDA), and the National Institute of Mental Health (NIMH). In 1975 ADAMHA established Treatment Assessment Research (TAR) as a separate research category specifically designed to study the relative safety and efficacy of various substances and procedures applied to human subjects. Examples include study of hyperbaric oxygen treatment for cognitive defects in the elderly and a study of intensive social casework and neuroleptic drugs in treatment of outpatient schizophrenia.

B. National Center for Health Services Research

This agency is authorized to undertake a broad range of research and evaluation activities pertaining to nearly all of health care delivery. A mixture of efficacy, safety, effectiveness, and cost information is often developed in its studies. For example, an investigation funded through the American College of Radiology focused on the efficacy of various x-ray procedures. The center uses "technical consensus" techniques similar to those of NIH. For example, a project funded through the American College of Cardiology studied "Optimal Electrocardiography."

C. Veterans Administration (VA)

Although the VA spends over 80 percent of its budget on direct care, the VA's Department of Medicine and Surgery has developed regulations, manuals, and circulars on the efficacy and safety of medical technologies and services. This department has a Research and Development Division involved in basic medical research, clinical trials, health services research, and rehabilitative engineering. The fiscal year 1976 research budget was $96 million. Examples of such studies include the famous drug treatment trials for hypertension, controlled trials of immune serum globulin for the prevention of posttransfusion hepatitis, and clinical trial of methadyl acetate and methadone as maintenance treatment for heroin addiction.

D. Department of Defense (DOD)

The Department of Defense supports a considerable amount of health-related research. The fiscal year 1976 research budget was $114 million. Study is directed toward those areas that affect the military, including clinical trials to test the efficacy and safety of medical technologies. Field medical care and evaluation systems, disease prevention, and field environment hazard reduction all have been subjects of efficacy studies.

Appendix C

Sources of National Data on Results of Effectiveness and Efficiency Studies

ɁɁɁɁɁɁɁɁɁɁɁɁɁɁɁɁɁɁɁɁɁɁɁɁɁ

Finding published or unpublished information on quality assurance data and methods is difficult. The strategies used for conducting a literature search for efficacy studies do not yield the same results for effectiveness and efficiency studies. Traditional indexes such as MEDLARS or the *Index Medicus,* though of exceptional value in identifying biomedical research studies, do not use the descriptors needed for most quality assurance studies. Moreover, much of the content of relevant quality assurance literature is not included in index data bases. Sources such as the publications of the National Center for Health Statistics, the transmittals of Professional Standards Review Organizations, and the bulletins and publications of the Joint Commission on Accreditation of Hospitals provide information on data and methods that are not indexed by the National Library of Medicine in MEDLARS. One approach to locating this information is to conduct a search based on the compilation date of the needed material. Two resources, organized by date of compilation, are:

- Literature before 1976

  See Williamson, J. *Improving Medical Practice and Health Care: A Bibliographic Guide to Information Management in Quality Assurance and Continuing Medical Education.* Cambridge, Mass.: Ballinger, 1978.

- Literature from 1976 and after

  See National Health Standards and Quality Information Clearinghouse (Health Standards and Quality Bureau, Health Care Financing Administration, Department of Health and Human Services, 6110 Executive Blvd., Rockville MD 20852 (301/881-9400).

Literature Before 1976

The bibliography recommended for locating quality assurance literature before 1976 is unique in several aspects. It is probably the most definitive compilation of quality assurance-related publications available covering the period 1900–1975. This book provides citations and abstracts for over 3,500 articles. Each article is coded to indicate its relevance to assessment of effectiveness of health care, efficiency of health care, and improvement of health care. Further, detailed descriptors are indexed to indicate the patient population, the health problem, the health care provider, and the care interaction (for example, diagnostic or therapeutic) featured in the article. Finally, detailed descriptors indicate quality assurance content in terms of assessment mechanisms or improvement modalities encompassed. The "concept coding" method of indexing used in this book will later be adopted by the PSRO Clearinghouse (now titled "National Health Standards and Quality Information Clearinghouse"). By this method it is possible to search any combination of codes delineating the concept that is the target of the search—for example, outcome assessment of diagnostic performance (Code 236) by general practitioners (Code 064) on geriatric patients (Code 047) suspected of having neoplastic disease (Code 137). If the reader's main emphasis in this search were on "effectiveness" of diagnostic care, Code 004 could be added; if emphasis were on efficiency (cost containment), Code 007 could be added. It is estimated that over 75 percent of the articles cited in this book would not be accessible by traditional medical literature indexes. The main reason is that most of the "jargon quality assurance terms" coded in this bibliography did not come into use until after the early 1970s. Further, it required expert quality assurance knowledge to recognize relevant articles that were written in traditional research terms. For example, "observer error" studies of the 1940s through 1960s provide examples of classic diagnostic validation investigations. Garfield's study wherein he had multiple radiologists read the same set of x rays (for which the findings were known as provided by autopsy) indicated the level of agreement and accuracy that can be achieved under ideal conditions (efficacy). In this case it was documented that, for reading chest films, 25 percent of known lesions will be missed by the average radiologist, regardless of the size or configuration of the lesion. This article has important implications for designing quality assessment projects. By reading articles coded 318, the reader can screen 164 such "observer error" studies on a wide variety of topics besides radiology. This applies to many other quality assurance topics, such as those related to successful attempts to achieve improvement of health care when serious problems were identified. For example, articles coded 333 include 247 published studies in which improvement impact was formally evaluated and achieved for a wide variety of topics. By taking a little time to become adept at using the code system in this bibliography, one can rather quickly identify a large number of relevant articles to facilitate not only the assessment of the effectiveness and efficiency of health care but most other quality assurance functions as well.

Literature from 1976

The National Health Standards and Quality Information Clearinghouse provides an invaluable ongoing reference index to the quality assurance (including cost containment) literature. Like Williamson's bibliography, this clearinghouse covers the traditional biomedical literature in MEDLARS/MEDLINE as well as considerable nonpublished sources, such as the information transmittals of the national PSRO program. Even pertinent information published in the *Federal Register* and lay press (for example, the *Wall Street Journal*) is indexed in this source. Much information related to quality assurance regulation and policy is important to be aware of in quality assurance activities. For example, changes in the quality assurance requirements of the Joint Commission on Accreditation of Hospitals are essential to understand. This clearinghouse facilitates access to such information long before it will be available in traditional medical journals. The search base of this source has been recently augmented to provide access to literature regarding long-term care that was previously very difficult to find. The coding index provides ready access to the jargon terms of quality assurance. (As much as one might decry jargon, it will always be a part of any specialized field, especially one that is growing as rapidly as quality assurance is.)

To obtain access to this clearinghouse, one can be put on its mailing list and receive, free of charge, the *Information Bulletin* published monthly, together with annual collations of the coded and indexed citations. Copies are often available in the offices of local PSROs and university libraries, if not local hospital libraries. The monthly *Bulletins* provide complete abstracts of all articles indexed. It is also possible to have special searches completed by the clearinghouse staff on request.

After these two sources (Williamson's bibliography and the PSRO Clearinghouse) have been searched and adequate information still has not been found, a limited final effort might be made to use the traditional indexes, such as the *Index Medicus,* MEDLARS, or MEDLINE, available in most university medical center libraries. The price will be the time required to screen a large proportion of articles that will be irrelevant in terms of information maturity and content. However, if a highly technical information need is the target of one's search, these computerized searches may prove of value.

Appendix D

Selected Bibliography on Learning Theory, Behavior, and Organizational Change[1]

ᛉᛈᛉᛈᛉᛈᛉᛈᛉᛈᛉᛈᛉᛈᛉᛈᛉᛈᛉᛈᛉᛈᛉᛈᛉᛈᛉᛈᛉᛈ

I. Application of Continuing Education to Competency Assessment, Performance, and Health Care Quality

AAMC Ad Hoc Committee on Continuing Medical Education. "Continuing Medical Education of Physicians: Conclusions and Recomendations." *Journal of Medical Education*, 1980, *55*, 149–157.

AAMC and Continuing Education Staff Development Services, Office of Academic Affairs, Veterans Administration. "Enhancing the Application of Adult Learning Principles to Continuing Education of Health Professionals." Phase A Report to the Veterans Administration. February 1980.

AAMC Division of Educational Resources and Programs. *Continuing Medical Education: Discussions Using Nominal Group Technique.* Washington, D.C.: AAMC, 1978.

AAMC Division of Educational Resources and Programs. *Continuing Medical Education: Results of Delphi Probe with Practitioners and Faculty.* Washington, D.C.: AAMC, 1978.

AAMC Division of Educational Resources and Programs. *Continuing Medical Education: An Analysis Tool for Examining Options.* Prepared by Pugh-Roberts Associates, Inc. Washington, D.C.: AAMC, 1978.

Brown, C. R., Jr. "The Continuing Education Component of the Bi-cycle Approach to Quality Assurance." In R.H. Egdahl and P. M. Gertman (Eds.), *Quality Health Care: The Role of Continuing Medical Education.* Germantown, Md.: Aspen Systems Corp., 1977.

Brown, C. R., Jr., and Fleisher, D. S. "The Bi-cycle Concept— Relating Continuing Education Directly to Patient Care." *New England Journal of Medicine,* 1971, *284,* Supplement.

Capital Systems Group, Inc. *Effect of Continuing Education on Physician Behavior. A Selected Annotated Bibliography.* Under Contract No. HSA 240-76-0018 BQA, DHEW. Rockville, Md.: DHEW, 1976.

Charters, A. N., and Blakely, R. J. *The Management of Continuing Learning: A Model of Continuing Education as a Problem-Solving Strategy for Health Manpower, Fostering the Growing Need to Learn. Monographs and Annotated Bibliography on Continuing Education and Health Manpower.* DHEW Pub. No. (HRA) 74-3112. Rockville, Md.: USDHEW/PHS, 1974.

Fleisher, D. S., Brown, C. R., Jr., Zeleznik, C., Escovitz, G. H., and

[1]For an extensive annotated bibliography on continuing medical education as related to quality assurance and behavioral change, see *Continuing Medical Education: A Selected Annotated Bibliography.* January 1979. Association of American Medical Colleges, Division of Educational Resources and Programs, 1 Dupont Circle NW, Washington DC 20036.

Omdal, C. "The Mandate Project: Institutionalizing a System of Patient Care Quality Assurance." *Pediatrics,* 1976, *57*(5), 775–782.

Gilbert, D. N., Eubanks, N. M., and Jackson, J. M. "The Effects of Monitoring the Use of Gentamicin in a Community Hospital." *Journal of Medical Education,* 1978, *53,* 129–134.

Hanlon, C. R., Egdahl, R. H., and Gertman, P. M. (Eds.). "Do Self-Assessment Methods of Continuing Medical Education Affect Quality of Patient Care?" In R. H. Egdahl and P. M. Gertman (Eds.), *Quality Health Care: The Role of Continuing Education.* Germantown, Md.: Aspen Systems Corp., 1977.

Mahan, J. M., Philips, B. U., and Constanzi, J. J. "Patient Referrals: A Behavioral Outcome of Continuing Medical Education." *Journal of Medical Education,* 1978, *53,* 210–211.

Menzel, H. "Innovation, Integration, and Marginality: A Survey of Physicians." *American Sociological Review,* 1960, *25,* 704–713.

Miller, G. E., Egdahl, R. H., and Gertman, P. M. (Eds.). "Challenges to Continuing Medical Education." In R. H. Egdahl and P. M. Gertman (Eds.), *Quality Health Care: The Role of Continuing Education.* Germantown, Md.: Aspen Systems Corp., 1977.

Monheit, A. C., Egdahl, R. H., and Gertman, P. M. (Eds.). "Benefit-Cost Aspects of Continuing Medical Education." In R. H. Egdahl and P. M. Gertman (Eds.), *Quality Health Care: The Role of Continuing Education.* Germantown, Md.: Aspen Systems Corp., 1977.

Nelson, A. R., Egdahl, R. H., and Gertman, P. M. (Eds.). "The Role of PSROs in Conducting and Evaluating Continuing Medical Education Programs." In R. H. Egdahl and P. M. Gertman (Eds.), *Quality Health Care: The Role of Continuing Education.* Germantown, Md.: Aspen Systems Corp., 1977.

Peterson, O. "The Impact of CME on the Quality of Care: What Are the Results?" In R. H. Egdahl and P. M. Gertman (Eds.), *Quality Health Care: The Role of Continuing Education.* Germantown, Md.: Aspen Systems Corp., 1977.

Stearns, N.S., Getchel, M.E., and Gold, R.A. "Continuing Medical Education in Hospitals: A Manual for Program Development." *New England Journal of Medicine,* 1971, *284*(20), Supplement.

Stein, L. S. *Your Personal Learning Plan: A Handbook for Physicians.* Chicago: Illinois Council on Continuing Medical Education, 1973.

Stein, L. S., Bordeaux, D., Furlong, N. K., and White, F. Z. *Patient-Problem Inventory—Planning CME Programs That Fit Staff Interests.* Chicago: Illinois Council on Continuing Medical Education, 1975.

Talley, R. C. "Effect of Continuing Medical Education on Practice Patterns." *Journal of Medical Education,* 1978, *53,* 602–603.

Whitney, M. A., and Caplan, R. M. "Learning Styles and Instructional Preferences of Family Practice Physicians." *Journal of Medical Education,* 1978, *53,* 684–685.

Williamson, J. W. *Improving Medical Practice and Health Care: A Bibliographic Guide to Information Management in Quality Assurance and Continuing Education.* Cambridge, Mass.: Ballinger, 1977.

II.   Learning Theory as Applied to Adult Professionals

Anderson, R. C., and Faust, G. W. *Education Psychology: The Science of Instruction and Learning.* New York: Harper & Row, 1973.

Bandura, A. *Principles of Behavioral Modification.* New York: Holt, Rinehart and Winston, 1969.

Bandura, A. *Social Learning Theory.* New York: General Learning Press, 1971.

Cawley, R. W. Z., Miller, S. A., and Milligan, J. N. "Cognitive Styles and the Adult Learner." *Adult Education,* 1976, *26*(2), 101–116.

Combs, A. W. (Ed.). *Perceiving, Behaving, Becoming: A New Focus for Education.* Washington, D.C.: Association for Supervision and Curriculm Development, 1962.

Della-Dora, D., and Blanchard, L. J. (Eds.). *Moving Toward Self-Directed Learning: Highlights of Relevant Research and of Promising Practices.* Alexandria, Va.: Association for Supervision and Curriculum Development, 1979.

Dewey, J. *Democracy and Education.* New York: Macmillan, 1951. (Originally published in 1916.)

Dewey, J. *The Quest for Certainty.* New York: Minton, Balch, 1929.

Dubin, S. S., and Okun, M. "Implications of Learning Theories for Adult Instruction." *Adult Education,* 1973, *24*(1), 3–19.

Gagné, R. M. *The Conditions of Learning.* (3rd ed.) New York: Holt, Rinehart and Winston, 1977.

Gagné, R. M., and Briggs, L. J. *Principles of Instructional Design.* (2nd ed.) New York: Holt, Rinehart and Winston, 1979.

Goulet, L. R., and Baltes, P. B. *Life-Span Developmental Psychology*. New York: Academic Press, 1970.

Gruber, H. E., and Weitman, M. "Self-Directed Study: Experiments in Higher Education." University of Colorado Behavior Research Laboratory Report #19. April 1962.

Guthrie, E. R. *The Psychology of Learning*. New York: Harper & Row, 1935.

Hilgard, E. R., and Bower, G. H. *Theories of Learning*. (4th ed.) Englewood Cliffs, N.J.: Prentice-Hall, 1975.

Houle, C. O. *The Design of Education*. San Francisco: Jossey-Bass, 1972.

Hull, C. L. *Principles of Behavior*. New York: Appleton-Century-Crofts, 1943.

Johnson, K. R., and Ruskin, R. S. *Behavioral Instruction: An Evaluative Review*. Washington, D.C.: American Psychological Association, 1977.

Johnson, R. B., and Johnson, S. R. *Assuring Learning with Self-Instructional Packages, or . . . up the Up Staircase*. Chapel Hill, N.C.: Self-Instructional Packages, 1971.

Keller, J. M. "Motivation and Instructional Design: A Theoretical Perspective." *Journal of Instructional Development*, Summer 1979, *2*, 26–34.

Kidd, J. R. *How Adults Learn*. New York: Association Press, 1973.

Knowles, M. S. *The Modern Practice of Adult Education: Andragogy versus Pedagogy*. New York: Association Press, 1974.

Knowles, M. S. *Self Directed Learning*. New York: Association Press, 1975.

Knox, A. B. "Life-Long Self-Directed Education." In *Fostering the Growing Need to Learn*. Rockville, Md.: DHEW Division of Regional Medical Programs, 1974.

Knox, A. B. "Professional Competence: Means and Ends." *Professional Engineer*, November 1975, pp. 49–52.

Knox, A. B. *Helping Adults to Learn*. Concept Paper No. 4. Washington, D.C.: Continuing Library Education Network and Exchange, 1976.

Knox, A. B. *Adult Development and Learning: A Handbook on Individual Growth and Competence in the Adult Years for Education and the Helping Professions*. San Francisco: Jossey-Bass, 1977.

Knox, A. B. "The Nature and Causes of Professional Obsolescence." Prepared for "The Evaluation of Continuing Education for Professionals: A Systems View," Lake Wilderness Continuing Education Center, September 13–15, 1978.

Knox, A. B. (Ed.). *New Directions for Continuing Education: Assessing the Impact of Continuing Education,* no. 3. San Francisco: Jossey-Bass, 1979.

Koffka, K. *The Growth of the Mind* (R. M. Ogden, trans.). London: Kegan Paul, Trench, Trubner, 1924.

Koffka, K. *Principles of Gestalt Psychology.* New York: Harcourt Brace Jovanovich, 1935.

Miller, H. L. *Teaching and Learning in Adult Education.* New York: Macmillan, 1964.

Monette, M. L. "The Concept of Educational Need." *Adult Education,* 1977, *27,* 116–127.

Pavlov, I. P. *Conditioned Reflexes.* London: Clarendon Press, 1927.

Penland, P. B. *Self-Planned Learning in America.* Pittsburgh: University of Pittsburgh Graduate School of Library and Information Sciences, 1977.

Piaget, J. *The Psychology of Intelligence.* New York: Harcourt Brace Jovanovich, 1950.

Rogers, C. R. *Freedom to Learn.* Columbus, Ohio: Merrill, 1969.

Rosenthal, T. L., and Zimmerman, B. J. *Social Learning and Cognition.* New York: Academic Press, 1978.

Skinner, B. F. *The Behavior of Organisms: An Experimental Analysis.* New York: Appleton-Century-Crofts, 1938.

Skinner, B. F. *The Technology of Teaching.* New York: Appleton-Century-Crofts, 1968.

Strike, K. "The Logic of Discovery Learning." *Review of Educational Research,* Summer 1975, *45,* 461–483.

Thorndike, E. L. *Educational Psychology.* New York: Lemcke and Buechner, 1903.

Tough, A. "Major Learning Efforts: Recent Research and Future Directions." Unpublished paper, 1977. Write: Department of Adult Education, Ontario Institute for Studies in Education, 252 Bloor Street West, Toronto, Ontario, M5S 1V6.

Tough, A. *The Adult's Learning Projects: A Fresh Approach to Theory and Practice in Adult Education.* (2nd ed.) Research in Education

Series No. 1. Toronto: Ontario Institute for Studies in Education, 1979.

Verner, C., and Davison, C. V. *Physiological Factors in Adult Learning and Instruction.* Tallahassee: Research Information Processing Center, Florida State University Department of Adult Education, 1971.

Wertheimer, M. "Untersuchung zur Lehre von der Gestalt, II." *Psychologische Forschung, 4,* 301–350. Translated and condensed as "Laws of Organization in Perceptual Forms." In W. D. Ellis, *A Source Book of Gestalt Psychology.* New York: Harcourt Brace Jovanovich, 1938.

Witkin, H. A., and others. "Field-Development and Field-Independent Cognitive Styles and Their Educational Implications." *Review of Educational Research,* Winter 1977, *47,* 1–64.

III.   Organizational Change

Beckhard, R. *Organization Development: Strategies and Models.* Reading, Mass.: Addison-Wesley, 1969.

Beckhard, R. "Strategies for Large System Change." *Sloan Management Review,* 1975, *16*(2), 43–55.

Beckhard, R., and Harris, R. T., "Management Structures and Processes in the Transition." In *Organizational Transitions: Managing Complex Change.* Reading, Mass.: Addison-Wesley, 1977.

Bennis, W. *Organization Development: Its Nature, Origins, Prospects.* Reading, Mass.: Addison-Wesley, 1969.

Daft, R. L. "System Influences on Organizational Decision Making: The Case of Resource Allocation." *Academy of Management Journal,* 1978, *21*(1), 6–22.

Delbecq. A., and Van de Ven, A. "A Group Process Model for Problem Identification and Program Planning." *Journal of Applied Behavioral Science,* 1971, *7*(4).

Derr, C. B. "Managing Organizational Conflict." *California Management Review,* 1978, *21*(2), 76–83.

Franklin, J. L. "Characteristics of Successful and Unsuccessful Organization Development." *Journal of Applied Behavioral Science,* 1976, *12*(4), 471–492.

Glaser, W. *Social Settings and Medical Organization: A Cross National Study of the Hospital.* New York: Atherton Press, 1970.

Greiner, L. E. "Patterns of Organization Change." In M. Dalton, P. R. Lawrence, and L.E. Greiner (Eds.), *Organizational Change and Development.* Homewood, Ill.:Irwin, Dorsey, 1970.

Hall, R. H., Hass, J. E., and Johnson, N. "Organizational Size, Complexity and Formalization." *American Sociological Review,* 1967, *32,* 903–913.

Katz, D., and Kahn, R. *The Social Psychology of Organizations.* New York: Wiley, 1978.

Klein, O. C. "Some Notes in the Dynamics of Resistance to Change: The Defender Role." In G. Watson (Ed.), *Concepts for Social Change.* Washington, D.C.: Cooperative Project for Educational Development, National Training Laboratories, National Education Association, 1967.

Levin, G., Roberts, E., Hirsch, G., Kligler, D., Wilder, J., and Roberts, N. *The Dynamics of Human Service Delivery.* Cambridge, Mass.: Ballinger, 1976.

Lindquist, J. *Strategies for Change.* Berkeley, Calif.: Pacific Sounding Press, 1978.

Mulder, M., and Wilke, H. "Participation and Power Equalization." *Organization Behavior and Human Performance,* 1970, *5.*

Ouchi, W. G. "The Relationship Between Organizational Structure and Organizational Control." *Administrative Science Quarterly,* 1977, *22*(1), 95–113.

Plovnick, M., Fry, R., Rubin, I., and Stearns, N. "Workshop: Improving Worker Coordination in Health Care Delivery." *Health Care Management Review,* Summer 1976, pp. 24–26.

Robbins, S. P. "'Conflict Management' and 'Conflict Resolution' Are Not Synonymous Terms." *California Management Review,* 1978, *21*(2), 67–75.

Roberts, E. B. "The Problems of Aging Organizations." *Business Horizons,* 1967, *10*(4), 51–58.

Robertson, L., Kosa, J., Heagarty, M., Haggerty, R., and Alpert, J. *Changing the Medical Care System: A Controlled Experiment in Comprehensive Care.* New York: Praeger, 1974.

Rubin, I., Plovnick, M., and Fry, R. "Initiating Planned Change in

Health Care Systems." *Journal of Applied Behavioral Science, 1974, 10,* 107–124.

Schein, E.H., *Process Consultation: Its Role in Organization Development.* Reading, Mass.: Addison-Wesley, 1969.

Schein, E. H., *Organizational Psychology.* (2nd ed.) Englewood Cliffs, N.J.: Prentice-Hall, 1970.

Schein, E. H. *Professional Education: Some New Directions.* Sponsored by the Carnegie Commission on Higher Education. New York: McGraw-Hill, 1972.

Schein, E. H. *Career Dynamics: Matching Individual and Career Needs.* Reading, Mass.: Addison-Wesley, 1978.

Shull, F. A., Delbecq, A. L., and Cummings, L. L. *Organizational Decision Making.* New York: McGraw-Hill, 1970.

Stearns, N. S., Bergan, T. A., Roberts, E. B., and Cavazos, L. F. "A Systems Intervention for Improving Medical School-Hospital Interrelationships." *Journal of Medical Education,* 1978, *53*(6), 464–472.

Student, K. R. "Managing Change: A Psychologist's Perspective." *Business Horizons,* 1978, *21*(6), 28–33.

Weisbord, M. R. "Why Organizational Development Hasn't Worked (So Far) in Medical Centers." *Health Care Management Review,* 1976, *1,* 18–31.

Weisbord, M. R., and others. "Three Dilemmas of Academic Medical Centers." *Journal of Applied Behavioral Science,* 1978, *14*(3), 284–304.

Appendix E

National Data on Cost-Benefit of Quality Assurance Activities[1]

⟩⟨

Examples

Brook, R., Williams, K., and Rolph, J. "Use, Costs, and Quality of Medical Services: Impact of the New Mexico Peer Review System. A 1971–1975 Study." *Annals of Internal Medicine,* 1978, *89*(2), 256–263.[2]

[1]Also see Appendix B, Section III—Reports of the Office of Technology Assessment, U.S. Congress.

[2]See also Brook, R., Williams, K., and Rolph, J. "Controlling the Use and Cost of Medical Services: The New Mexico Experimental Medical Care Review Organization. A Four Year Case Study." *Medical Care,* 1978, *16*(9) (Supplement).

Reports data based on a New Mexico study and concludes that (1) utilization review had no demonstrable impact on hospital use and (2) peer review produced no net dollar savings. However, this report indicates that peer review did improve the quality of ambulatory care through large reductions in unnecessary injections.

Brook, R., and Williams, K. "Effect of Medical Care Review on Use of Injections. A Study of the New Mexico Experimental Medical Care Review Organization." *Annals of Internal Medicine*, 1976, *85*(4), 509–515.[3]

Cites data on the improvement in proper use of injections among physicians in HMOs as a result of peer review activities.

Assessing Quality in Health Care: An Evaluation. Institute of Medicine, National Academy of Sciences. November 1976.

Reports that (1) MCEs may have caused improvement in quality; (2) reliable, generalizable assessments have not yet been made; (3) evidence is not yet available that hospital concurrent review is (cost) effective; and (4) most ambulatory claims review programs considered in the study yielded dollar reductions in submitted claims more than adequate to pay for the costs of review. The report included recommendations for more targeted review, more efforts to evaluate federal and privately sponsored quality assurance programs by comparing quality of care with and without quality review programs, fewer but better-designed and better-evaluated MCEs, and use of uniform data elements for all health settings. Most of these recommendations have been implemented. For copies of this report, write:
IOM Publication 74-04
Institute of Medicine
National Academy of Sciences
2101 Constitution Avenue
Washington DC 20418

[3]See also Lohr, K., Brook, R., and Kaufman, M. A. "Quality of Care in the New Mexico Medicaid Program (1971–1975). The Effect of the New Mexico Experimental Medical Care Review Organization on the Use of Antibiotics for Common Infectious Diseases." *Medical Care*, 1980, *18* (1) (Supplement).

Effect of PSROs on Health Care Costs: Current Findings and Future Evaluations. U.S. Congress, Congressional Budget Office. June 1979. 77 pages.

Suggests that PSROs may not be cost-effective, since they may not be as effective in reducing utilization by populations other than Medicare, Medicaid (for example, veterans and private patients). Copies of this report are available from the U.S. Congress, Office of the Budget, Washington, DC.

Report to the Congress on the PSRO Program. U.S. General Accounting Office. June 16, 1980.

Suggests that PSROs are, in fact, becoming cost-effective and that some of the contentions made in the earlier CBO report are unfounded. Copies of this report are available from the U.S. General Accounting Office, 441 G Street NW, Washington, DC.

PSRO Impact on Medical Care Services in Selected Areas of the United States. Potomac, Md.: American Association of PSROs. February 1, 1980.

Presents data indicating substantial utilization reduction in the private sector due to PSRO activities. For copies of this report, write: American Association of PSROs, 11325 Seven Locks Road, Suite 214, Potomac MD 20854.

Annual Reports to the Congress on the PSRO Program. Health Care Financing Administration, Office of Research, Demonstrations and Statistics.[4]

Reports findings for fiscal year 1977, published in April 1978, as follows: No aggregate PSRO effect on utilization variables studied, although some organizations were

[4]For a description of a complete evaluation plan for PSRO, see Baum, M., McMenamin, A., and Rudor, M., *Program Evaluation Plan: Professional Standards Review Organizations.* Office of Research, Evaluation, and Planning, DHEW. September 22, 1975.

associated with lower (favorable) utilization, while others reflected higher (unfavorable) rates; some decreases (favorable) in average length of stay for Medicare patients; no favorable impact on Medicaid patients; and MCEs completed through full cycle demonstrated effective identification and correction of problems.

Reports finding for fiscal year 1978, published in 1979, as follows: The national program saved the Medicare program an estimated $5 million more than it cost to administer the reviews.

Reports findings for fiscal year 1979, published in May 1980,[5] as follows: The national program saved the Medicare program an estimated $21 million more than it cost to administer the reviews. The largest savings were demonstrated in the Northeast, where PSROs have been in operation longer.

For copies of these annual reports, write: Office of Research, Demonstrations and Statistics, Health Care Financing Administration, U.S. Department of Health and Human Services, Baltimore, MD 21235.

[5]*Health Care Financing Research Report: Professional Standards Review Organization, 1979 Program Evaluation.* Published by Health Care Financing Administration, Office of Research, Demonstrations and Statistics. HCFA Pub. No. 03041, May 1980.

References

Acton, J. P. *Evaluating Public Programs to Save Lives: The Case of Heart Attacks.* Pub. No. R-950-RC. Santa Monica, Calif.: Rand Corporation, 1973.

Acton, J. P. *Measuring the Social Impact of Heart and Circulatory Disease Programs: Preliminary Framework and Estimates.* Pub. No. R-1697-NHL. Santa Monica, Calif.: Rand Corporation, 1975.

Acton, J. P. *Measuring the Monetary Value of Lifesaving Programs.* Pub. No. P-5675. Santa Monica, Calif.: Rand Corporation, 1976.

American Board of Medical Specialties. *1978–1979 Annual Report.* Chicago: American Board of Medical Specialties, 1979.

American Heart Association, Subcommittee on Risk of Heart Attack and Stroke. *Stroke Risk Handbook—Estimating Risk of Stroke in Daily Practice.* New York: American Heart Association, 1974.

Becker, M. H., Drachman, R. H., and Kirscht, J. P. "A New Approach to Explaining Sick-Role Behavior to Low-Income Populations." *American Journal of Public Health,* 1974, *64,* 205–216.

Becker, M. H., and Maiman, L. A. "Sociobehavioral Determinants of Compliance with Health and Medical Care Recommendations." *Medical Care,* 1975, *12,* 10–24.

Beckhard, R. *Organization Development: Strategies and Models.* Reading, Mass.: Addison-Wesley, 1969.

Bennis, W. G. *Organization Development: Its Nature, Origins and Prospects.* Reading, Mass.: Addison-Wesley, 1969.

Bertram, D. A., and Brooks-Bertram, P. A. "The Evaluation of Continuing Medical Education: A Literature Review." *Health Education Monographs,* 1977, *5*(4), 330–362.

Bouchard, R. E., and Tufo, H. M. "Problem-Oriented Approach to Practice: II. Development of the System Through Audit and Implication." *Journal of the American Medical Association,* 1977, *236,* 502–505.

Brook, R. H. *Quality of Care Assessment: A Comparison of Five Methods of Peer Reviews.* DHEW Pub. No. (HRS)74-3100. Rockville, Md.: Department of Health, Education and Welfare, 1974.

Brook, R. H., Williams, K. N., and Rolph, J. E. *Quality of Medical Care Assessment Using Outcome Measures: An Overview of the Method.* Pub. No. HEW R-2021/1. Santa Monica, Calif.: Rand Corporation, 1978. Also published in *Medical Care,* 1978, *16* (Supplement).

Brown, C. R., and Fleisher, D. S. "The Bi-Cycle Concept: Relating Continuing Education Directly to Patient Care." *New England Journal of Medicine,* 1971, *284* (Supplement).

Bunker, J., Barnes, B., and Mosteller, F. *Costs, Risks, and Benefits of Surgery.* New York: Oxford University Press, 1977.

California Medical Association/California Hospital Association. *Educational Patient Care Audit Manual.* San Francisco: California Medical Association/California Hospital Association, 1975.

Cochrane, A. *Effectiveness and Efficiency: Random Reflections on Health Services.* London: Nuffield Provincial Hospital Trust, 1972.

Codman, E. A. *A Study in Hospital Efficiency.* Boston: Thomas Todd, 1916.

Commission to Study Social Insurance and Unemployment. *Hear-*

ings Before the Committee on Labor, House, 64th Congress, April 6 and 11, 1916. Washington, D.C.: U.S. Government Printing Office, 1918.

Cooper, B. S., and Rice, D. P. "The Economic Cost of Illness Revisited." DHEW Pub. No. (SSA)76-11703. *Social Security Bulletin,* February 1976.

Dawson, W. H. *Social Insurance in Germany, 1883–1911.* New York: Scribner's, n.d.

Delbecq, A., Van de Ven, A., and Gustafson, D. *Group Techniques for Program Planning: A Guide to Nominal Group and Delphi Process.* Glenview, Ill.: Scott, Foresman, 1975.

Drexler, A., Yenney, S. L., and Hohman, J. "OD: Coping with Change." *Hospitals,* 1977a, *51*(1), 58–60.

Drexler, A., Yenney, S. L., and Hohman, J. "OD Team Building: What It's All About." *Hospitals,* 1977b, *51*(2), 99–104.

Farrington, J. F., Felch, W. C., and Hare, R. L. "Quality Assessment and Quality Assurance." *New England Journal of Medicine,* 1980, *303(3),* 153–156.

Fetter, R. B., Mills, R. E., Riedel, D. C., and Thompson, J. D. "The Application of Diagnostic Specific Cost Profiles to Cost and Reimbursement Control in Hospitals." *Journal of Medical Systems,* 1977, *1,* 137–149.

Fetter, R. B., Shin, Y., Freeman, J. L., Averill, R. F., and Thompson, J. D. "Case Mix Definition of Diagnostic-Related Groups." *Medical Care,* 1980, *18* (Supplement).

Fetter, R. B., Thompson, J. D., and Mills, R. E. "A System for Cost and Reimbursement Control in Hospitals." *Yale Biology Journal,* 1976, *49,* 123–126.

Fink, R., Shapiro, S., and Lewison, J. "The Reluctant Participant in Breast Cancer Screening Programs." *Public Health Reports,* 1968, *83,* 479–490.

Flach, E. *Participation in Case Finding Programs for Cervical Cancer: Administrative Report, Cancer Control Program.* U.S. Public Health Service. Washington, D.C.: Government Printing Office, 1960.

Galen, R. S., and Gambino, S. R. *Beyond Normality: The Predictive Value and Efficiency of Medical Diagnoses.* New York: Wiley, 1975.

Gifford, R. H., and Feinstein, A. R. "A Critique of Methodology in Studies of Anti-Coagulant Therapy for Acute Myocardial Infarction." *New England Journal of Medicine,* 1969, *280,* 351–357.

Gonnella, J. S., Cattani, J. A., Louis, D. Z., and others. "Use of Outcome Measure in Ambulatory Care Evaluation." In G. A. Giebink, N. H. White, and E. S. Short (Eds.), *Ambulatory Medical Care Quality Assurance.* La Jolla, Calif.: La Jolla Health Science Publications, 1977.

Haefner, D. P., and Kirscht, J. P. "Motivational and Behavioral Effects of Modifying Health Beliefs." *Public Health Reports,* 1970, *85,* 478–484.

Hiatt, H. H. "Protecting the Medical Commons: Who Is Responsible?" *New England Journal of Medicine,* 1975, *293,* 235–241.

Hochbaum, G. M. *Public Participation in Medical Screening Programs: A Socio-Psychological Study.* PHS Pub. No. 572. Washington, D.C.: U.S. Government Printing Office, 1958.

Hu, T., and Sandifer, F. H. *Synthesis of Cost of Illness Methodology.* Prepared for the National Center for Health Services Research, Office of the Assistant Secretary for Health, Public Health Service, Department of Health and Human Services (Contract No. 233-79-3010), 1981.

Institute of Medicine. *Advancing the Quality of Health Care: Key Issues and Fundamental Principles.* Washington, D.C.: National Academy of Sciences, 1974.

Inui, T. S., Yourtee, E. L., and Williamson, J. W. "Improved Outcomes in Hypertension After Physician Tutorials: A Controlled Trial." *Annals of Internal Medicine,* 1976, *84,* 646-651.

Jessee, W. F. "Physician Competence and Compulsory Continuing Education: Are They Compatible?" *Journal of Community Health,* 1977a, *1,* 291–295.

Jessee, W. F. "Quality Assurance Systems: Why Aren't There Any?" *Quality Review Bulletin,* 1977b, *3*(11), 16–18ff.

Joint Commission on Accreditation of Hospitals. "New Quality Assurance Standard of the JCAH." *Quality Review Bulletin,* 1979, *5,* 4–5.

Kannel, W. B., Wolf, P., and Dawker, T. R. "Hypertension and Cardiac Impairments Increase Stroke Risk." *Geriatrics,* 1978, *33* (9), 71–83.

Kaplan, S. H., and Greenfield, S. "Criteria Mapping: Using Logic in Evaluation of Processes of Care." *Quality Review Bulletin*, 1978, *4*, 3–9.

Kegeles, S. S. "A Field Experiment to Change Beliefs and Behavior of Women in an Urban Ghetto." *Journal of Health and Social Behavior*, 1969, *10*, 115.

Kessner, D. M., Kalk, C. E., and Singer, J. "Assessing Health Quality: The Case for Tracers." *New England Journal of Medicine*, 1973, *288*, 189–194.

Kidd, J. R. *How Adults Learn*. New York: Association Press, 1973.

Knox, A. B. *Adult Development and Learning: A Handbook on Individual Growth and Competence in the Adult Years for Education and the Helping Professions*. San Francisco: Jossey-Bass, 1977.

Lawrence, P. R., and Lorsch, J. W. *Organization and Environment*. Homewood, Ill.: Irwin, 1969.

Lawrence, P. R., Weisbord, M. R., and Charms, M. P. "The Organization and Management of Academic Medical Centers: A Summary of Findings." Unpublished report, Organization Research and Development, Block, Petrella and Associates, 1974.

Laxdal, D. E., Jennett, P. A., Wilson, T. W., and Salisbury, G. M. "Improving Physician Performance by Continuing Medical Education." *Canadian Medical Association Journal*, 1978, *118*, 1051–1058.

Lilienfeld, A. M. *Foundations of Epidemiology*. New York: Oxford University Press, 1976.

Lowe, J. A. "PASport." *Quality Review Bulletin*, 1977a, *3*, 20–24.

Lowe, J. A. "The Quality Assurance Monitor and MCE Studies." Paper presented at a workshop on alternative approaches to MCE studies, Chicago, 1977b.

MacDonald, C. J. "Protocol-Based Computer Reminders, the Quality of Care and the Non-Perfectibility of Man." *New England Journal of Medicine*, 1975, *295*, 1351–1355.

MacMahon, B., and Pugh, T. F. *Epidemiology: Principles and Methods*. Boston: Little, Brown, 1970.

Mills, D. H. "Report of the California Medical Insurance Feasibility Study." Unpublished report, California Medical Association/California Hospital Association, 1977.

Mills, R., Fetter, R. B., Riedel, D. C., and Averill, R. "AUTOGRP:

An Interactive Computer System for the Analysis of Health Care Data." *Medical Care,* 1976, *14,* 603–615.

Mushlin, A. I. "An Experimental Mechanism for Quality Assurance in a Pre-Paid Group Practice." In *Proceedings of the Group Health Institute.* Washington, D.C.: Group Health Association of America, 1974.

Mushlin, A. I., and Appel, P. A. "Quality Assurance in Primary Care: A Strategy Based on Outcome Assessment." *Journal of Community Health,* 1978, *3,* 292–305.

Mushlin, A. I., and Appel, P. A., "Testing an Outcome-Based Quality Assurance Strategy in Primary Care." *Medical Care,* 1980, *18*(5), Supplement.

National Center for Health Statistics. *Vital and Health Statistics.* No. 1. Washington, D.C.: Health Resources Administration, Department of Health, Education, and Welfare, 1976.

Numbers, R. L. *Almost Persuaded: American Physicians and Compulsory Health Insurance, 1912–1920.* Baltimore and London: Johns Hopkins University Press, 1978.

Office of Technology Assessment. *Assessing the Efficacy and Safety of Medical Technologies.* Pub. No. 052-003-00593-0. Washington, D.C.: U.S. Government Printing Office, 1978.

Ogilvie, R., and Ruedy, J. "An Educational Program in Digitalis Therapy." *Journal of the American Medical Association,* 1972, *222,* 50–55.

Pliskin, N., and Taylor, A. "General Principles: Cost-Benefit and Decision Analysis." In J. Bunker and others (Eds.), *Costs, Risks, and Benefits of Surgery.* New York: Oxford University Press, 1977.

Querido, A. *The Efficiency of Medical Care.* Leiden: Stenfert Kroese, 1963.

Roemer, M. I. "Government's Role in American Medicine—A Brief Historical Survey." *Bulletin of the History of Medicine,* 1945, *18,* 146–168.

Rubin, L., and Kellogg, M. A. "The Comprehensive Quality Assurance System." In G. A. Giebink, N. H. White, and E. S. Short (Eds.), *Ambulatory Medical Care Quality Assurance.* La Jolla, Calif.: La Jolla Health Sciences Publications, 1977.

Sackett, D. L., and Haynes, R. B. *Compliance with Therapeutic Regimens.* Baltimore: Johns Hopkins University Press, 1976.

Sanazaro, P. J., and Williamson, J. W. "End Results of Medical Care: A Provisional Classification Based on Reports by Internists." *Medical Care,* 1968, *6*(2), 123–190.

Sanazaro, P. J., and Worth, R. M. "Concurrent Quality Assurance in Hospital Care: Report of a Study by Private Initiative in PSRO." *New England Journal of Medicine,* 1978, *198,* 1171–1177.

Schein, E. H. *Process Consultation: Its Role in Organization Development.* Reading, Mass.: Addison-Wesley, 1969.

Schein, E. H. *Organizational Psychology.* (2nd ed.) Englewood Cliffs, N.J.: Prentice-Hall, 1970.

Schein, E. H. *Professional Education: Some New Directions.* Profile series sponsored by the Carnegie Commission on Higher Education, No. 10. Berkeley, Calif.: McGraw-Hill, 1972.

Smith, W. M. "Treatment of Mild Hypertension: Results of a Ten Year Intervention Trial." *Circulation Research,* 1977, *40* (Supplement 1), 98–105.

Smith, W. M. "Hypertension—Effectiveness of Early Treatment in Preventing Sequelae." Paper presented at seminar on Preventive Interventions in the Practice of Medicine, Rancho Mirage, Calif., March 15, 1979.

Stamler, J., and Epstein, F. H. "Coronary Heart Disease: Risk Factors as Guides to Preventive Actions." *Preventive Medicine,* 1972, *1,* 27–48.

Starfield, B. H. "Achieving Coordination in Primary Care." Paper presented at meeting of the Ambulatory Pediatric Association, New York, April 1978.

Starfield, B. H., Simborg, D. W., Horn, S. D., and Yourtee, S. A. "Continuity and Coordination in Primary Care: Their Achievement and Utility." *Medical Care,* 1976, *14,* 625–636.

Stason, W. B., and Weinstein, M. C. "Allocation of Resources to Manage Hypertension." *New England Journal of Medicine,* 1977, *296,* 732–739.

Terris, M. "An Early System of Compulsory Health Insurance in the United States, 1798–1884." *Bulletin of the History of Medicine,* 1944, *15,* 433–444.

Thompson, J. D., Fetter, R. B., and Mross, C. D. "Case Mix and Resource Use." *Inquiry,* 1973, *17,* 300–312.

Tufo, H. M., Bouchard, R. E., Rubin, A. S., Twitchell, J. C., Van

Buren, H. C., Weed, L. B., and Rothwell, M. "Problem-Oriented Approach to Practice." *Journal of the American Medical Association,* 1979, *238,* 414–417, 502, 505.

U. S. Department of Health, Education, and Welfare, Health Care Financing Administration, Health Standards and Quality Bureau. *PSRO Program Manual.* Washington, D.C.: U. S. Government Printing Office, 1974.

Veterans Administration Cooperative Study Group on Antihypertensive Agents. "Effects of Treatment on Morbidity in Hypertension. Results in Patients with Diastolic Blood Pressure Averaging 115 Through 129 mm Hg." *Journal of the American Medical Association,* 1967, *202,* 1028–1034.

Veterans Administration Cooperative Study Group on Antihypertensive Agents. "Effects of Treatment on Morbidity in Hypertension. Part 2: Results in Patients with Diastolic Blood Pressure Averaging 90 Through 114 mm Hg." *Journal of the American Medical Association,* 1970, *213,* 1143–1152.

Veterans Administration Cooperative Study Group on Antihypertensive Agents. "Effects of Treatment on Morbidity in Hypertension. Part 3: Influence of Age, Diastolic Pressure, and Prior Cardiovascular Disease; Further Analysis of Side-Effects." *Circulation,* 1972, *45,* 991–1004.

Weisbord, M. R. "A Mixed Model for Medical Centers: Changing Structure and Behavior." In J. Adams (Ed.), *Theory and Method in Organization Development: An Evolutionary Process.* Arlington, Va.: NTL, Institute for Applied Behavioral Science, 1974.

Weisbord, M. R. "Why Organization Development Hasn't Worked (So Far) in Medical Centers." *Health Care Management Review,* 1976, *1,* 18–31.

Williams, P. *The Purchase of Medical Care Through Fixed Periodic Payment.* New York: National Bureau of Economic Research, 1932.

Williamson, J. W. *Assessing and Improving Health Care Outcomes: The Health Accounting Approach to Quality Assurance.* Cambridge, Mass.: Ballinger, 1978.

Williamson, J. W., Alexander, M., and Miller, G. E. "Continuing Education in Patient Care Research: Physician Response to Screening Test Results." *Journal of the American Medical Association,* 1967, *201,* 938–942.

Williamson, J. W., Aronovitch, S., Simonson, L., Ramirez, C., and Kelly, D. "Health Accounting, an Outcome-Based System of Quality Assurance: Illustrative Application to Hypertension." *Bulletin of the New York Academy of Medicine*, 1975, *51* (6), 727–738.

Young, W. W., Swinkola, R. B., and Hutton, M. D. "Assessment of the AUTOGRP Patient Care Classification System." *Medical Care*, 1980, *18*, 228.

Index

A

Acton, J. P., 21, 66, 101, 129
Adult learning: bibliography on, 119–122; principles of, and improved health care, 45–46, 47, 77
Alcohol, Drug Abuse, and Mental Health Administration, 109
Alexander, M., 38, 42, 136
Alpert, J., 123
American Association for Labor Legislation, Committee on Social Insurance of, 7
American Association of Foundations of Medical Care, 11
American Association of Professional Standards Review Organizations, 11
American Board of Medical Specialties, 3, 129
American College of Cardiology, 109
American College of Radiology, 109
American Federation of Labor, 7
American Heart Association, 65, 129
American Medical Association, 92–93
American Socialist Party, 7
American Society of Internal Medicine, 3
Anderson, R. C., 119
Appel, F. A., 37, 134
Association of American Medical Colleges, 116–117

B

Baltes, P. B., 120
Bandura, A., 119
Barnes, B., 23, 130
Baum, M., 127n
Becker, M. H., 44–45, 129–130
Beckhard, R., 43, 122
Behavior modification, and improved health care, 45, 47
Benefits: of quality assurance, 83–84; type of, and efficacy, 26–27
Bennett, W., 9, 11
Bennis, W. G., 43, 44, 122, 130
Bergan, T. A., 124
Berk, A., 99–100
Bertram, D. A., 47, 77, 80, 130
Bi-cycle, for effectiveness and efficiency, 36
Blakely, R. J., 117
Blanchard, L. J., 119
Blue Cross, forerunner of, 7
Bordeaux, D., 119
Bouchard, R. E., 45, 130, 135–136

138